Advance praise f ▌▌▌▌▌ *Health*

"Dr. Koenig's lifelong rese     ...ccessfully bridges the chasm between health and well-being on the one side and religion and spirituality on the other. In so doing, we are given scientifically based guidelines that allow us to be happier and more fulfilled. I highly recommend *Medicine, Religion and Health* and thank Dr. Koenig for all of his outstanding contributions."

— Herbert Benson, M.D., director emeritus, Benson-Henry Institute for Mind Body Medicine at Massachusetts General Hospital and Mind-Body Medical Institute Associate Professor of Medicine, Harvard Medical School

"Here Harold Koenig provides, as few can, an expert review of findings at the interface between medicine and religion, clear discussion of what the evidence means, and practical recommendations for integrating scientific and spiritual care. This concise volume is valuable both as an accessible introduction to the literature for lay readers and as a thoughtful guide for professionals interested in improving their practice."

— John R. Peteet, M.D., associate professor of psychiatry, Harvard Medical School, Brigham and Women's Hospital, and Dana-Farber Cancer Institute

"Koenig's book is a concise, articulate, and compelling story of the interplay between spirituality, religiousness, and health. The general public will find it fascinating and informative reading, while doctors and medical students will find it essential for their understanding of, and compassionate caring for, their patients."

— Robert G. Brooks, M.D., M.A. (Theol.), M.B.A., associate dean for health affairs and professor of family medicine and rural health, Florida State University College of Medicine

DISCARD

"This is an essential book not only for physicians but for anyone involved in a health care discipline—professionals, patients, and families alike . . . The book goes beyond research by offering clear, concise, and helpful recommendations for how to address religious and spiritual issues and how to utilize the expertise of all professionals within the healthcare team in partnering with patients to provide the best and most compassionate care possible. It is a volume not only important for professionals; it is one that would serve medical, nursing, chaplaincy, and other health care professionals well in their training."

—Sue Wintz, chaplain, St. Joseph's Hospital and Medical Center and the Barrow Neurological Institute, Phoenix, Arizona

"I very much enjoyed reading this book and have no hesitation recommending it for any person interested in the religion/health interaction. Those experienced in the field will find it refreshing to read, those new to the field will find it a useful initial source for future in-depth study, and those unaware of the field may find it intriguing and stimulating. It also could make a nice gift for those not particularly interested in the field as it may draw their attention to important issues they were not aware of and that may have a significant impact."

—Ronald C. Hamdy, M.D., F.R.C.P., F.A.C.P., editor-in-chief, *Southern Medical Journal* and professor of medicine and Cecile Cox Quillen Chair, Geriatric Medicine and Gerontology College of Medicine, East Tennessee State University

# Medicine, Religion, *and* Health

# Templeton Science and Religion Series

In our fast-paced and high-tech era, when visual information seems so dominant, the need for short and compelling books has increased. This conciseness and convenience is the goal of the Templeton Science and Religion Series. We have commissioned scientists in a range of fields to distill their experience and knowledge into a brief tour of their specialties. They are writing for a general audience, readers with interests in the sciences or the humanities, which includes religion and theology. The relationship between science and religion has been likened to four types of doorways. The first two enter a realm of "conflict" or "separation" between these two views of life and the world. The next two doorways, however, open to a world of "interaction" or "harmony" between science and religion. We have asked our authors to enter these latter doorways to judge the possibilities. They begin with their sciences and, in aiming to address religion, return with a wide variety of critical viewpoints. We hope these short books open intellectual doors of every kind to readers of all backgrounds.

**Series Editors:** J. Wentzel van Huyssteen & Khalil Chamcham
**Project Editor:** Larry Witham

# Medicine, Religion, *and* Health

WHERE SCIENCE *&* SPIRITUALITY MEET

Harold G. Koenig, M.D.

TEMPLETON FOUNDATION PRESS

WEST CONSHOHOCKEN, PENNSYLVANIA

Templeton Foundation Press
300 Conshohocken State Road, Suite 670
West Conshohocken, PA 19428
www.templetonpress.org

*Templeton Foundation Press helps intellectual leaders and others learn about science research on aspects of realities, invisible and intangible. Spiritual realities include unlimited love, accelerating creativity, worship, and the benefits of purpose in persons and in the cosmos.*

Designed and typeset by Gopa and Ted2, Inc.

Library of Congress Cataloging-in-Publication Data

Koenig, Harold George.
  Medicine, religion, and health : where science and spirituality meet / Harold G. Koenig.
    p. ; cm. — (Templeton science and religion series)
    Includes bibliographical references and index.
    ISBN-13: 978-1-59947-141-9 (pbk. : alk. paper)
    ISBN-10: 1-59947-141-8 (pbk. : alk. paper)
  1. Medicine—Religious aspects. 2. Health—Religious aspects. I. Title. II. Series.
  [DNLM: 1. Spiritual Therapies. 2. Mental Healing. 3. Mind-Body Relations (Metaphysics) 4. Religion and Medicine. 5. Spirituality. WB 880 K78m 2008]
    BL65.M4K648 2008
201'661—dc22
2008008159

Printed in the United States of America

08 09 10 11 12 13 10 9 8 7 6 5 4 3 2 1

To Martha Haley

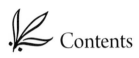 Contents

Introduction                                            3

Chapter  1  Terms of the Debate                         9

Chapter  2  Medicine in the Twenty-first Century       21

Chapter  3  From Mind to Body                          37

Chapter  4  Religion and Health                        54

Chapter  5  Mental Health                              68

Chapter  6  The Immune and Endocrine Systems           82

Chapter  7  The Cardiovascular System                  96

Chapter  8  Diseases Related to Stress and Behavior   113

Chapter  9  Longevity                                 129

Chapter 10  Physical Disability                       146

Chapter 11  Clinical Applications                     156

Chapter 12  Final Thoughts                            172

Appendix    Further Resources                         175

Notes                                                 195

Index                                                 227

Medicine, Religion, *and* Health

# Introduction

MRS. HARRIS DIED yesterday at the age of one hundred and one. She was living in a nursing home, but her family says that she was alert to the very end. In her final days, as she had throughout her life, she tried to console and encourage family members and friends—even from her sickbed. She pointed out their good qualities. She expressed what a joy it was to see him or her and what a special future was ahead for each. Her family said that she was singing a religious hymn when her voice became weaker, her breathing became slower, and then finally stopped. Mrs. Harris left behind a slight smile on her face, a smile her family had become used to whenever she was deeply content.

When Mrs. Harris had turned one hundred, she was asked the secret for her long life. She quickly responded that it was her faith, her family, and that she didn't drink or smoke, in that order. And the order was important, she emphasized.

Many doctors have known a "Mrs. Harris," as I often have, and while we can imagine meeting her in any state or city, in a hospital or a nursing home, she stands for a real-life benchmark of health, both physical and mental. Her kind of story, in which people tie their beliefs and their behaviors to health, is the primary topic of this book. Mrs. Harris is based on my two and a half decades of experience with patients and research subjects and I will use her "story" throughout the book to demonstrate the types of encounters that I have had. Mrs. Harris' responses illustrate the very real life experiences that many, many people report—experiences that are often ignored by health professionals.

The following pages cover a lot of ground, not all of which is flat and level. Our information is still incomplete on the effects of religion and spirituality on mental and physical health. The discussion of this topic is also new in modern medicine. As a result, there are many opinions on what we really know in this field, what should be done about it, and how. I will point out where there is controversy on a particular finding or application. But I will also argue for a connection between religion and health when the preponderance of the evidence, along with common sense and logical reason, supports that link. This book will, therefore, not be short on controversy, and I hope that will intrigue the reader.

I have organized the material in four steps, building one upon another. I begin by defining the terms *religion* and *spirituality* and showing how research on their relationship to health and medicine has dramatically grown and will become crucial to a possible future health-care crisis. After this, I present the case that religion and spirituality can indeed affect health in a scientifically detectable way. In other words, the psychological, social, and religious aspects of human life can be shown to affect the physical body. Finding the mechanisms or pathways by which religion affects health is central to helping scientists and clinicians understand how and why religion is related to health.

Once I have presented the case that such pathways are plausible, I will probe more deeply into six specific areas of human health possibly affected by religious involvement. These are areas where someone like Mrs. Harris was very fortunate, thanks to a good outlook on life, healthy habits, and a strong body. The six areas are mental health, immune and endocrine functions, cardiovascular function, stress and behavior-related disease, mortality, and physical disability. Once we are reasonably clear on how religion may affect health, and explore the scientific evidence supporting such claims, I will examine the application of this knowledge to treating patients in clinical settings. An appendix will conclude this volume by listing resources for further study of religion, spirituality, and health.

Each of the chapters that follow will survey past and current research, but each will also contain a central point that I wish to argue, or at least leave open for discussion. In chapter 1, for example, I will show that opinions diverge wildly on the definitions of the terms *religion* and *spirituality*. The term spirituality is a broad one that allows people to provide their own definitions. This inclusiveness is helpful in clinical settings where doctors want to be sensitive to the wide range of beliefs of individuals. But, in research, these terms must be more precisely defined for objective study of their impact on health, and that precision is what I will advocate. Otherwise, I will often use *religion* and *spirituality* interchangeably, referring to the same side of human experience.

In chapter 2, I hypothesize that this rapidly growing area of research will become more important in the future as more strains are placed on health care, especially demographic and financial stressors. The aging populations in developed countries and the rapidly increasing costs of health care around the world are the two forces driving this increasing strain. I also foresee an increased role for faith communities to provide health care, not only in hospitals but also in terms of health education, social support, and long-term care.

The third and fourth chapters attempt to show that psychological and social factors influence the health of the physical body. Not long ago this was a controversial idea. In a 1985 editorial, for example, Marcia Angell, former editor-in-chief of the *New England Journal of Medicine*, stated that, "our belief in disease as a direct reflection of mental state is largely folklore."[1] Since that editorial was written, many studies published in some of the best science journals in the world have proven her wrong. Today, we have a rapidly growing field called *psychoneuroimmunology* —closely related to "psychosomatic medicine"—that looks at how mental and social experiences can impact aspects of physical health.

My basic thesis in chapters 5 through 10 is that religion has the potential to influence both mental and physical health. In chapter 5, I look at religion and mental health covering such areas of human experience as depression, anxiety, and positive emotions. Chapter 6 examines associations between religion, the immune system, and endocrine functions, with a focus on relationships in different age groups and in different diseases such as fibromyalgia, metastatic breast cancer, and HIV/AIDS. In chapter 7, I explore religion's effects on the heart and circulatory system: cardiovascular reactivity, blood pressure, autonomic and carviovascular rhythms, and on behaviors such as diet, exercise, and cigarette smoking that affect those physiological functions. Chapter 8 examines the clinical consequences of religious involvement on rates of coronary artery disease and outcomes following cardiac surgery, as well as on common maladies such as cancer, age-related memory decline, Alzheimer's disease, and diabetes.

In chapter 9, I review several studies of large populations in the United States, Europe, and Asia that examine the relationship of religious involvement to longevity. This is a much disputed area, and I will look at the complexities of interpreting such studies but will argue that while the evidence for religion and longer life is only moderate in strength, it has a huge public health impact. Chapter 10 looks at what I think is perhaps the most important question—not how long we live, but the quality of our lives and the ability to physically carry out activities that make life worth living. Long-term illnesses in later life take an emotional toll and have an impact on the ability to work, on social life, and on recreational activities. Here I will also discuss the relationship between religion and disability in young persons with acquired health problems due to premature disease, accidents, or war.

The book ends with applications of this new research. In chapter 11, I argue that the research findings have implications for health professionals, especially recognition of the many ways that religious beliefs can influence health care, patient compliance, and medical decisions.[2] These are important reasons why health professionals should pay attention to the spiritual needs of patients and be aware of the boundaries and limitations in this area. Here I describe how and when spirituality can be integrated into patient care and what are the likely consequences. Finally, the appendix provides summaries of (a) key original research studies on religion and health, (b) review papers of the religion–health research, (c) books on religion, spirituality, and health for researchers, clinicians, and the general public, and (d) Internet sites and academic centers of activity in religion, spirituality, and health where further resources can be located.

The primary goal of *Medicine, Religion, and Health* is to explore and make sense of some of the recent research on religion, spirituality, and health, and to do this in a relatively concise and readable format. Because of this focus, a more thorough discussion of theological issues has not been attempted. Bear in mind, however, that this research has raised a number of serious theological concerns that also need to be addressed. A comprehensive scientific review and theological discussion of the religion–health connection will be covered in a much larger volume, which is now in preparation.[3] For now, however, let us explore the latest scientific evidence linking religion, spirituality, and health, and explore what that means for doctors, patients, and those who are healthy and want to stay that way.

When Mrs. Harris said that the reasons for her long life were her faith, her family, and her avoidance of alcohol and cigarettes—in that order—she was trying to communicate something about the keys to health and well-being that she had learned during her long and satisfying life. She will speak to us a few more times in the pages ahead as we delve more deeply into this topic.

## CHAPTER 1
## Terms of the Debate

WHENEVER I GIVE a public talk on religion and health issues, I try to avoid one thorny topic in particular: defining the differences between the words *religion* and *spirituality*. This can easily alienate a significant proportion of the audience because each of us has our own definitions for these words, which we hold onto quite dearly. In this book, however, I have the luxury of spending some time exploring these terms in depth. Establishing definitions now for how I am using these terms will help the reader understand what the research means and will assist medical professionals in applying the findings to their clinical practices.

Without crystal-clear definitions, research on religion, spirituality, and health is not possible. For example, if a relationship is discovered between "spirituality" and longevity, what does that mean? The word *longevity* is widely understood as meaning years of life, and this can be calculated precisely by knowing birth and death dates. In contrast, there is no universal agreement on the more nebulous term *spirituality*. But if a relationship between spirituality and longevity is found, we need to know what this thing "spirituality" is in order to understand what exactly is related to a long life span.

We also need to know how spirituality differs from other psychosocial concepts, such as psychological well-being, altruism, forgiveness, humanism, social connectedness, and quality of life. Spirituality must be unique and different from everything else, a completely separate phenomenon, which can then be examined in its relationship to health. Our task in conducting research is to quantify how spiritual the person is (determine the extent or degree that the person is spiritual) and describe in what ways he or she is spiritual. This is absolutely necessary in order to determine how spirituality is related to health.

To focus on these distinctions, this chapter compares four concepts—religion, spirituality, humanism, and positive psychology—with particular attention paid to spirituality, since this is such a commonly used term today. The meaning of the term *spirituality* has broadened in recent years to include positive psychological concepts such as meaning and purpose, connectedness, peacefulness, personal well-being, and happiness. According to researchers Christian Smith and Melinda Denton, "The very idea and language of 'spirituality,' originally grounded in the self-disciplining faith practices of religious believers, including ascetics and monks, then becomes detached from its moorings in historical religious traditions and is redefined in terms of subjective self-fulfillment."[1] This new version of spirituality has evolved to include not only aspects of life that have nothing to do with religion but often excludes religion entirely, as in the statement "I'm spiritual, not religious." This can make spirituality indistinguishable from concepts that are secular.

There are both positive and negative consequences to broadening of the term *spiritual*. In this book, which focuses on research, I will argue that we need to reinstate a sharper definition of *spirituality* that retains its historical grounding in religion. Nevertheless, I will admit that the broadening of the term has a valuable clinical application. As we shall see, then, spirituality can be profitably used in two different ways, more narrowly in research and more broadly for patient care. Before presenting a definition for spirituality, however, I will first define religion and then review attempts by others to define spirituality as something unique and different from religion.

## RELIGION

*Religion* may be defined as a system of beliefs and practices observed by a community, supported by rituals that acknowledge, worship, communicate with, or approach the Sacred, the Divine, God (in Western cultures), or Ultimate Truth, Reality, or nirvana (in Eastern cultures). Religion usually relies on a set of scriptures or teachings that describe the meaning and purpose of the world, the individual's place in it, the responsibilities of individuals to one another, and the nature of life after death. Religion typically offers a moral code of conduct that is agreed upon by members of the community, who attempt to adhere to that code.

Religious activity may be public, social, and institutional ("organizational" religiosity) or can be private, personal, and individual ("nonorganizational" religiosity). Organizational religiosity involves attending religious services, meeting as a group at other times for prayer or scripture study, or involvement with others in church-related activity, such as evangelism, fund-raising, financial giving or church-related volunteering (I use the term *church* here for succinctness and ease of reading. What is intended is church, synagogue, mosque, or temple). Nonorganizational religiosity refers to religious activity that is done alone and in private, such as praying or communicating with God at home, meditating, reading religious scriptures, watching religious television or listening to religious radio, or performing private rituals such as lighting candles, wearing religious jewelry, and so forth.

Although religious practices (public and private) often reflect how deeply religious a person is, this is not always the case. To fill this gap, there is a dimension of religion that has to do with the importance or centrality of religion in life. This has been called *subjective religiosity* and is measured by researchers with self-ratings of religious importance or overall religiousness. There is also a motivational dimension of religion that is closely related to subjective religiosity but that asks *why* the person is religiously involved. What motivates the person to be religious? Is religion sought for its own value, i.e., as an end in itself ("intrinsic" religiosity), or is it being used as a means to some other end that is ultimately more important, such as social position or financial gain ("extrinsic" religiosity)? Although the organizational, nonorganizational, subjective, and motivational aspects of religion are considered by some to be the most salient, there are many other dimensions, including religious belief or orthodoxy, religious knowledge, religious coping, religious quest (or seeking), religious history, religious maturity, and religious well-being.[2]

In addition to its traditional form, religion also has a nontraditional shape, since it can be used to describe a wide array of groups guided by common beliefs and rituals. These include astrology, divination, witchcraft, invoking of spirits, spiritism, and a variety of indigenous, folk, or animistic rituals and practices related to the supernatural. Under my definition, therefore, religion is a unique domain with multiple dimensions that can be measured, quantified, and examined in relation to health and medical outcomes. Most high-quality research on religion, spirituality, and health actually ends up measuring religion, even many studies that use the term *spirituality* in the title or when discussing results.

## SPIRITUALITY

I propose that, for pragmatic reasons there should be two definitions of the term *spirituality*: one for conducting research and studying the relationship between spirituality and health and one for applying what has been discovered to the care of patients. But first, how is *spirituality* usually defined? It has become a popular and accommodating term, especially in secular academic circles, because its vagueness, broadness, and dependence on self-definition. This term can include everybody, even the nonreligious. Below are several definitions for the term by experts in the field. The first three are definitions developed by health professionals

involved in the *clinical care* of patients, which helps to explain why
they are so broad and inclusive:

: The definition [of *spirituality*] is based in every person's inher-
ent search for ultimate meaning and purpose in life. That
meaning can be found in religion but may often be broader
than that, including a relationship with a god/divine figure or
transcendence; relationships with others; as well as spirituality found in nature, art, and rational thought.[3]

: The concept of spirituality is found in all cultures and societ-
ies. It is expressed in an individual's search for ultimate meaning through participation in religion and/or belief in God,
family, naturalism, rationalism, humanism, and the arts. All of
these factors can influence how patients and health care professionals perceive health and illness and how they interact
with one another.[4]

: Spirituality is a complex and multidimensional part of the
human experience. It has cognitive, experiential, and behavior aspects. The cognitive or philosophic aspects include the
search for meaning, purpose, and truth in life and the beliefs
and values by which an individual lives. The experiential and
emotional aspects involve feelings of hope, love, connection,
inner peace, comfort and support. These are reflected in the
quality of an individual's inner resources, the ability to give and
receive spiritual love, and the types of relationships and connections that exist with self, the community, the environment
and nature, and the transcendent (e.g., power greater than
self, a value system, God, cosmic consciousness). The behavior aspects of spirituality involve the way a person externally
manifests individual spiritual beliefs and inner spiritual state.
Many people find spirituality through religion or through a
personal relationship with the divine. However, others may
find it through a connection to nature, through music and the
arts, through a set of values and principles or through a quest
for scientific truth.[5]

Notice how these definitions of *spirituality* include meaning and purpose, inner peace and comfort, connection with others, support, feelings of wonder, awe, or love, and other healthy, positive terms. The definitions also make it very clear that spirituality does not have to involve religion—i.e., it can be completely secular. Here, *spirituality* is defined by however a person chooses to define it, but it always means something good—something that almost anyone would want to associate with. While such broad definitions work well in clinical practice, they cause havoc when trying to conduct research. The difficulty of measuring such a concept and examining its relationship to health, especially mental health, should be obvious.[6] I will say more about this later.

Peter C. Hill and Ken Pargament, well-known researchers in this area, define *spirituality* in a more unique way to help distinguish it from other related concepts. They argue that in the United States and elsewhere there is

a polarization of religiousness and spirituality, with the former representing an institutional, formal, outward, doctrinal, authoritarian, inhibiting expression and the latter representing an individual, subjective, emotional, inward, unsystematic, freeing expression. . . . [S]pirituality can be understood as a search for the sacred, a process through which people seek to discover, hold on to, and, when necessary, transform whatever they hold sacred in their lives. . . . This search takes place in a larger religious context, one that may be traditional or non-traditional. . . . The sacred is what distinguishes religion and spirituality from other phenomena. It refers to those special objects or events set apart from the ordinary and thus deserving of veneration. The sacred includes concepts of God, the divine, Ultimate Reality, and the transcendent, as well as any aspect of life that takes on extraordinary character by virtue of its association with or representation of such concepts. . . .[7]

In another article, Pargament further explains:

> I see spirituality as a search for the sacred. It is, I believe, the
> most central function of religion. It has to do with however
> people think, feel, act, or interrelate in their efforts to find,
> conserve, and if necessary, transform the sacred in their lives.
> Let me say a bit more about the sacred. In the Oxford Eng-
> lish Dictionary, the sacred is defined as the holy, those things
> "set apart" from the ordinary, worthy of reverence. The sacred
> encompasses concepts of God, the divine, the transcend-
> ent, but it is not limited to notions of higher powers. It also
> includes objects, attributes, or qualities that become sancti-
> fied by virtue of their association with or representation of
> the holy.[8]

David J. Hufford, an authority in the medical humanities who
holds a Ph.D. in folklore and folk life from the University of Pennsylvania, makes the following observation:

> The odd thing about the inconsistency, vagueness and worry
> by investigators over these terms [religion and spirituality] is
> that they do have consistent, concise meanings in ordinary
> speech, and they relate to one another in a perfectly ordinary
> way. We are accustomed to pairs of words such as learning
> and education or health and medicine, where the former
> word identifies a broad domain and the second word refers
> to an institutional aspect of that domain. . . . Not all learning
> happens in schools and not all health behavior takes place in
> clinics or hospitals. Spirituality and religion stand in the
> same relation. Spirituality refers to the domain of spirit(s):
> God or gods, souls, angels, kjinni, demons. In short, this is
> what was once called the supernatural (and still is by many
> English speakers). When spirituality refers to something else
> it is by metaphorical extension to other intangible and invis-
> ible things. . . .[9]

In attempting to generalize his observations, Hufford specifically comments on the applicability of what he is saying to Eastern traditions.

> It is sometimes suggested that spirit(s) comprise a Western category and that some traditions, Buddhism being an often cited example, lack the concept. But as long as the concept is kept simple in definition this is not a valid criticism. The concept of reincarnation in Buddhism may not involve a concept analogous to the Western idea of a soul in some of its versions, but it nonetheless does involve something invisible and intangible that is a kind of essence of the person that reincarnates. . . . It is sometimes claimed that Buddhism is not a religion, sometimes defended on the basis that it is not theistic. Even apart from the fact that much of Buddhist beliefs and practice around the world DOES involve gods, clearly Buddhism is an institution organized around such ideas as reincarnation and Nirvana and it teaches practices that affect the intangible part of the human, the part that progresses or degenerates, that approaches enlightenment and Nirvana.[10]

In the end, Hufford defines *spirituality* simply as "personal relationship to the transcendent" and *religion* as "the community, institutional aspects of spirituality."[11]

## RECOMMENDED DEFINITION

For research purposes, my definition of *spirituality* comes closest to Hufford's. To facilitate measurement as a unique and distinct concept, I believe we should return the definition of *spirituality* to its origins in religion, whether traditional or nontraditional.[12] In its historical usage, the term *spirituality* has its roots in the patristic era and later spiritual thought derived from monastic life, the mendicants, the late Middle Ages, Luther, Ignatius, Teresa, and John of the Cross. Because the word *spirituality* has historically been associated with religion or the supernatural and involves religious language, I argue that, to call something spiritual, it must have some connection to religion.

Bear in mind that my definition of *religion* above includes non-traditional religious expressions. These include astrology, divination, witchcraft, folk traditions, or other indigenous healing practices that involve invisible spirits and spiritual forces that are outside of the individual yet are often practiced with others as part of a community with a set of beliefs, rituals, and moral code. My definition of the word *religion* also includes personal and private kinds of beliefs and activities not tied to organized or institutional worship. Religion also includes searching for or seeking the Sacred or transcendent, as the religious quest dimension would measure. However, if there is no connection with either religion or the supernatural, then I would not call a belief, practice, or experience spiritual. I would call it humanistic. An apt definition of the latter would be the following:

> Humanism is a broad category of active ethical philosophies that affirm the dignity and worth of all people, based on the ability to determine right and wrong by appeal to universal human qualities—particularly rationalism. Humanism is a component of a variety of more specific philosophical systems, and is also incorporated into some religious schools of thought. Humanism entails a commitment to the search for truth and morality through human means in support of human interests. In focusing on the capacity for self-determination, Humanism rejects transcendental justifications, such as a dependence on faith, the supernatural, or divinely revealed texts.[13]

In the area of spirituality, another important distinction must be made. When someone speaks of inner peace, connection with others, purpose and meaning, beliefs and values, feelings of wonder, awe, or love, forgiveness, gratitude, comfort, support, and other quasi-indicators of good mental health, this is not spirituality itself but the *result* of devoutly practiced spirituality. These good things are the consequences of living a spiritual life, *not spirituality itself*. Whether spiritual sources are more likely than secular sources to result in these positive psychological states is something that research must determine; spirituality cannot be defined by its consequences. Simply defining spirituality as good mental heath and including mental health indicators as part of the measures of spirituality precludes any ability to actually study the relationship between spirituality and mental health. To do so with a measure of spirituality contaminated by questions tapping positive psychological states or traits is called "tautology," a kind of circular reasoning that involves correlating a concept with itself. This kind of research always finds a positive correlation between spirituality and mental health (and often with physical health as well, due to the close connection between mental and physical health). Thus, when spirituality is used in research to study health, it cannot be defined in terms of positive or healthy psychological or social states.[14]

In the care of patients, however, it is not necessary to define spirituality as rigorously as when conducting scientific research. In clinical settings, it is more useful to define *spirituality* as broadly as possible so that all patients have an opportunity to have their spiritual needs addressed (in whatever way they define those spiritual needs). Some patients may not view themselves as religious but may nevertheless be searching for greater meaning outside themselves or struggling with existential concerns. Those may not be neatly categorized into psychological or social problems that lie within the expertise of mental health professionals or social workers. Again, definitions of *religion* and *spirituality* do not have to be as crisp and distinctive in clinical environments as they do in research settings.

Many patients may not understand the differences that academic health professionals are now making between religion and spirituality. In research that asked 838 patients to categorize themselves as either religious, spiritual, both, or neither, close to 90 percent indicated that they were both religious and spiritual.[15] Thus, a term is needed that everyone—religious and nonreligious alike—can relate to. It is not surprising, then, that definitions of *spirituality* by health professionals that I describe above are so broad and inclusive. But this will not do in research, which seeks to be discriminating, exclusive, and reductionistic in order to determine exactly what is affecting what.

Having different definitions for *spirituality* depending on the setting (research versus clinical) is not without potential problems, however. What if research shows that religious types of spirituality are related to better health, whereas nonreligious spirituality is either unrelated to health or related to worse health outcomes? In studies performed thus far, the finding is that greater *religious* involvement is related to better health—with the research strongest for mental health and less solid (but still impressive) for physical health. In the studies that I will review in later chapters, we will see that most of the existing research lumps "spiritual-but-not-religious" patients into the nonreligious group, the one that appears to be doing worse than religious patients. These studies seldom examine the spiritual-but-not-religious patients separately from other nonreligious patients. But the idea that spiritual-but-not-religious types may actually do worse is still a distinct possibility. What then? Should clinicians be asked to support the beliefs of spiritual-but-not-religious patients whose belief system may be having no effect or possibly even negative effects on health?

I believe the overall goal of the clinician is to find common ground with all patients, and that means not trying to change beliefs, but rather trying to support beliefs that help patients cope. Using spirituality in its broadest definition, then, makes sense in clinical practice (see chapter 11).

## Conclusions

Finding the proper distinctions between religion, spirituality, humanism, and other psychosocial concepts is especially important for research that wants to identify the exact causes of better health and medical outcomes. The vague use of the word *spirituality* has become a methodological problem in this sort of research, compounded when measures are contaminated by mental health indicators. A new clarity and specificity will be needed to advance knowledge in this field of study. I believe we must start by holding to a research definition of *spirituality* that has some connection to religion or the supernatural. If no such connection is found, then some other descriptive term should be used, such as a *humanistic* or some other already established psychological term. For clinical purposes, however, it is probably best to use a broader definition of *spirituality* that includes religious and nonreligious types and is self-defined by patients themselves. We want as many patients as possible to have an opportunity to have their spiritual needs identified and addressed, however they understand them.

One thing for sure, since experts are unlikely to agree on a common definition of *spirituality* in the near future, it is important that researchers, writers, and speakers on this topic make explicit how they are using this term.

## CHAPTER 2

# Medicine in the Twenty-first Century

"DOCTOR, YOU SAY that I have terminal cancer and there isn't any more that you can do for me. You say that I have two or three months left. What happens then? I'm afraid of the pain and suffering ahead. I'm afraid that I haven't been a good person. I'm afraid that God doesn't love me, since my prayers for healing have gone unanswered. I'm afraid of where I'm going after I die. I'm afraid of leaving my daughter and son, and never seeing them again. I'm afraid, doctor, I'm so afraid."

For people who face a serious illness, these are often the most pressing concerns. Increasingly, both health professionals and the medical system must tackle such personal inquiries. Furthermore, they will soon be confronted with a possible future health-care crisis, driven inexorably now by financial pressures and an aging population.

The research and policy questions abound. Should health professionals take more seriously the spiritual concerns of patients, and can this be a way to approach individual patients more compassionately as well as to strengthen and reform the health-care system? If these spiritual concerns are taken into account, what might health care look like thirty years from now? If health-care systems in the coming decades can no longer function as they have in the past, what are the options and how might faith communities be helpful?

Our approach to such policy questions will help determine the quality of care that patients receive in the future. This chapter will try to answer two policy questions in particular. First, does research confirm that health professionals should be looking at the spiritual needs of patients? And, second, how important might this be in responding to a health-care crisis should this develop in the future? To answer these, I will briefly describe the current situation of research on religion, spirituality, and health and discuss how this research is being applied to the clinical care of patients. Next, I will give an overview of medicine and health care in the twenty-first century, looking both at areas of crisis and also at new resources that may be found in religious organizations and faith communities.

The good news is that research on religion, spirituality, and health is advancing as never before, even though most doctors are still not trained to talk to patients about these issues. The bad news is in the headlines every day: the health-care systems of the world are headed for troubled times, unless we find innovative solutions.

## Religion-Health Research

By the year 2000, the number of studies examining the relationship between some aspect of religion, spirituality, and health or health care had ballooned to nearly 1,200 (about 70 percent were on mental health and 30 percent on physical health).[1] Since then, hundreds more studies have been published. Thus, it is safe to say that over one thousand research studies have quantitatively examined relationships between religion, spirituality, and health, many reporting positive findings.

This research has prompted at least three consensus conferences partially supported by the National Institutes of Health (NIH) to review the research and come up with recommendations for methodological advances and future studies.[2] William R. Miller, chair of the latest NIH working group, concluded, "Substantial empirical evidence points to links between spiritual/religious factors and health in U.S. populations. . . ."[3] While it is clear that many of the hundreds of studies published in the scientific literature have serious methodological flaws, not all of the studies do, and the critique of earlier research may have been overstated.[4] Furthermore, the quality of religion-health studies has increased substantially since the last NIH conference in 2002, with investigators responding to and correcting many of the concerns voiced about prior research.

While the field of religion, spirituality, and health is in its infancy and much research is needed to verify (or dispel) earlier findings, a lot of outstanding work has already been done. There is good reason to begin implementing some of what is already known in clinical practice.

## CLINICAL PRACTICE APPLICATIONS

Not all of the reasons for addressing spiritual issues in clinical practice depend on research that definitively demonstrates that religion influences health. The application is for very practical reasons: Many patients are religious, have religious beliefs and traditions related to health, and have health problems that often give rise to spiritual needs. Religious beliefs will frequently influence the kind of health care that patients wish to receive. Those beliefs affect how patients cope with illness and derive meaning and purpose when feeling bad physically or unable to do the things they used to do that give them joy and pleasure. Such beliefs help patients maintain hope and motivation toward self-care in the midst of overwhelming circumstances. Patients, particularly when hospitalized, may be isolated from their religious communities, and, because spiritual needs often come up during this time, health-care providers must recognize and address those needs. Religious beliefs can also influence medical decisions, conflict with medical treatments, and influence patients' compliance with treatments prescribed. The patient's involvement in a religious community can affect the support and monitoring he or she receives after discharge. In summary, there are many reasons for clinicians to discuss religious or spiritual issues with patients, learn to identify spiritual needs, and refer patients to health professionals trained to address those needs.[5]

The need for training to integrate spirituality into patient care has been increasingly recognized within medical education. In 1992, only three medical schools offered courses on religion, spirituality, and medicine. By 2006, over one hundred of the 141 medical schools in the U.S. and Canada had such courses (70 percent of which are required).[6] Unfortunately, most physicians in practice today have no such training. In a recent nationwide survey of a random sample of over one thousand U.S. physicians of all specialties, only about 10 percent of physicians indicated they routinely talked to patients about these issues.[7] Those data are consistent with reports by patients. Only 10 to 20 percent of patients report that a physician *ever* asked about spiritual issues.[8] As leaders in health care, physicians ought to be responsible for ensuring that spiritual needs likely to affect medical decisions and health outcomes are addressed.

Evidence that even the spiritual needs of dying patients are often unmet and the adverse effect of this on quality of life has recently been reported. Balboni and colleagues surveyed 230 patients with advanced cancer who had failed to respond to first-line chemotherapy.[9] These patients were being cared for at some of the best medical-care systems in the world, including Yale University Cancer Center in New Haven, Connecticut, and Memorial Sloan-Kettering Cancer Center in New York City. This study, conducted by Harvard Medical School researchers, had patients rate on a one to five scale to what extent either their religious community or the medical system supported their spiritual needs (from "not at all" to "completely supported"). One out of every two patients (47 percent) said that spiritual needs were minimally or not at all met by their religious community. Nearly three-quarters (72 percent) said that spiritual needs were minimally or not at all met by the medical system (i.e., doctors, nurses, or chaplains). Patients who indicated that their spiritual needs were being met reported significantly higher quality of life. In fact, of nine factors known to influence quality of life, degree of spiritual support was the second strongest predictor.

Unfortunately, there are not enough chaplains employed by hospital organizations to screen all patients or address the spiritual needs that are present, nor do community clergy have the time or expertise to meet those needs. Chaplains see only about 20 percent of hospitalized patients in the U.S. today.[10] In the current environment of intense competition among hospitals to survive financially, chaplain services are often the first to be downsized or eliminated.[11] The results of a survey on patient satisfaction that involved 1,732,562 patients representing 33 percent of all hospitals in the United States and 44 percent of all hospitals with more than one hundred beds found that satisfaction with the emotional and spiritual aspects of care received one of the lowest ratings of all clinical-care indicators. At the same time, it was one of the areas rated the highest for need of quality improvement.[12] This is a major reason why physicians, nurses, social workers, and other health professionals need to get more involved. There are not enough chaplains in hospital settings to see all the patients, so health professionals need to identify patients with the most pressing spiritual needs and get them connected to the few chaplains that are available to address them. However, there is resistance to doing so, particularly among physicians.

## Physician Attitudes

Despite what we know about the spiritual needs of patients and their relationship to health and well-being, few health professionals are addressing them. Most of what we know about the behaviors and attitudes of health professionals comes from studies of physicians. As noted earlier, only one in ten doctors regularly addresses spiritual issues with patients. So how do physicians in general feel about becoming more involved in this area?

Most physicians (over 90 percent) acknowledge that spiritual factors are an important component of health and the majority (70 to 82 percent) say that this can influence the health of the patient.[13] Furthermore, 85 percent of physicians say that they should be aware of the patient's religious/spiritual beliefs, and 89 percent indicate that they have a right to inquire about those beliefs.[14] Despite these positive attitudes, however, physicians are reluctant with patients about spiritual issues or to taking a spiritual history.

Doctors respond differently to such questions when asked about patients being treated in different settings, such as in outpatient clinics, acute hospital environments, or hospice-type circumstances. Depending on setting, 31 to 74 percent of physicians feel that they should take a spiritual history. They are more likely to do this as the patient's medical condition becomes more severe.[15] The best data on physicians' attitudes toward taking a spiritual history come from Curlin and colleagues' national survey of physicians mentioned earlier (see note 7 in this chapter). In that study, 55 percent said it was usually or always appropriate for physicians to inquire about patients' religious/spiritual beliefs, whereas 45 percent said it was usually or always *inappropriate* to do so. Thus, there appears to be a gap between what physicians feel they need to know and what they feel is appropriate to do in order to gather that information.

Interestingly, as the Curlin and colleagues survey shows, the strongest predictor of whether or not a physician addresses spiritual issues with patients has nothing to do with the patient's condition. Rather, it depends on how religious or spiritual the physician is. Common sense in this era of patient-centered medicine dictates that it ought to be the characteristics of the patient that determine whether spiritual matters are addressed, not the characteristics of the physician. Having insufficient time is also not the most common reason for ignoring patients' spiritual needs.[16] Moreover, recent data, again supplied by Curlin and associates, suggest that physicians who say that time is a barrier to addressing spiritual needs are actually more likely to talk with patients about these issues than physicians who don't indicate that time is a problem.

In my opinion, physicians should *make* time to inquire about spiritual issues that may directly or indirectly influence the health and health care of patients. A brief screening spiritual history takes only a few minutes. There are other interventions that physicians may choose to do beyond simple inquiry, although they will depend on the comfort level of the physician. Such interventions involve supporting the religious/spiritual beliefs of the patient and, if requested, praying with patients. In the national survey of physicians by Curlin and colleagues, 73 percent of physicians said that they often or always encouraged the patient's own religious/ spiritual beliefs and practices (versus sharing their own religious beliefs with patients). Other research (now twenty years old) suggests that about one-third of physicians have at some point in their careers prayed with a patient, with the vast majority of these physicians reporting that it had benefited the patient.[17] While many physicians feel that it is appropriate for them to pray with patients *if the patient asks*, only a small percentage (6 to 30 percent) say that it is appropriate for physicians to initiate prayer with patients.[18] Most physicians feel uncomfortable about initiating prayer with patients, particularly physicians who are not religious themselves. In general, though, physicians feel that the sicker the patient is, the more appropriate it is to inquire about spiritual matters or pray with him.

In summary, most physicians (and probably other health professionals as well) recognize the importance and value of patients' spiritual beliefs in the health of those patients and feel that they need to know about these beliefs. However, when asked specifically about what they are doing and what is appropriate to do, few physicians actively assess or address spiritual issues or are open to doing more in this area. Several forces on the horizon, though, are likely to change the attitudes of health-care professionals and health-care systems toward addressing spiritual issues and working with religious communities.

## HEALTH CARE IN THE TWENTY-FIRST CENTURY

Demographic, political and financial factors are now coalescing to create a "perfect storm" in health-care environments of the United States and other countries. The impact of that storm will become more and more evident during the next fifty years. Consider the following remarks made by Douglas Holtz-Eakin, director of the U.S. Congressional Budget Office, at a Health Care Congress sponsored by the *Wall Street Journal* and *CNBC* in Washington, DC:

> There are no silver bullets. There is no single item—technology, disease management, tort law—that is likely to prove to be the answer to aligning incentives, providing high-quality care at reasonable costs, and financing it in a way that's economically viable. . . . Rising health-care costs represent *the central domestic issue* at this time. [Over the next fifty years, if nothing is done] the cost of Medicare and Medicaid will rise from 4 percent of the gross domestic product to 20 percent—the current size of the entire federal budget.[19]

Those are pretty strong words. Why is this situation so?

### Demographic Changes

Because of advances in health care and public health practices that are extending longevity, the U.S. population and the populations of other developed countries around the world are beginning to age. The trend toward greater longevity after age sixty-five, together with lower birth rates in developed countries, has combined to increase the proportion of older persons in the population. In 2000, 35 million of the 282 million persons in the U.S. were over age sixty-five. According to the U.S. Census middle-series projections, by 2040, the population over age sixty-five will exceed 77 million, and those over age eighty-five will exceed 14 million.[20] These population estimates, however, do not take into account such potentially life-extending medical advances as genetic therapy or stem-cell research. More generous (and likely accurate) estimates for 2040 put the U.S. population over age sixty-five at 87 million and the population over age eighty-five at nearly 18 million.[21] Such numbers could easily overwhelm our health system's ability to provide health care to aging baby boomers (the 70–80 million persons born between 1945 and 1964).

### Costs of Health Care

The cost of health care is also skyrocketing. The rate of increase far exceeds the rate of inflation (8.4 percent per year from 2001 to 2004,[22] compared to 2.9 percent per year for inflation from 2000 to 2006[23]). This rise is occurring even before the first wave of baby boomers turn age sixty-five in 2011. According to the Center for Medicare and Medicaid Services, the cost of Medicare in 1993 was $148 billion, in 2000 was $225 billion, in 2002 was $267 billion, and in 2004 was $306 billion; for Medicaid, it was $77 billion in 1993, $118 billion in 2000, $148 billion in 2002, and $171 billion in 2004.[24] By 2014, the projected yearly cost of Medicare is a staggering $747 billion, and for Medicaid it is $355 billion. If one includes $193 billion of federal expenses due to the Medicaid SCHIP expansion, the result is a whopping $1.3 trillion in federal expenditures for health care in 2014 alone.[25] It is pretty clear that we will soon have a major health-care funding crisis on our hands.

Some experts have ventured to make predictions for what things will look like in 2040. Ed Schneider, dean of the Leonard Davis School of Gerontology, Andrus Gerontology Center, at the University of Southern California in Los Angeles, laid some out in the journal *Science* in February 1999.[26] If current levels of support for aging research, disease prevention, and treatment are sustained at the present rate, Schneider predicted that acute-care hospitals will become more and more like intensive-care units. Hospital stays will become shorter as efforts to save costs become more urgent. As soon as acutely ill patients are stabilized, they will be discharged to nursing homes to recover.

Nursing homes, on the other hand, will begin to resemble acute-care hospitals. Their patient acuity level will rise. Waiting lists for nursing homes will grow as facilities become packed with recovering patients. Most older adults with chronic health conditions will have no other choice but to remain at home, be cared for by their families, and receive medical treatment as outpatients. This includes most of the projected 14 million persons with Alzheimer's disease and the millions more with severe disability needing twenty-four-hour care.[27] Schneider concludes by stating that, "If they do not have relatives, significant others, or friends to take care of them, we may face the gruesome prospect of poor, disabled, homeless older Americans living out the end of their lives on city streets and in parks" (see note 26).

Other developed countries will have it far worse than the United States. The United States is ranked only thirty-third among developed countries in terms of its aging population.[28] The United Nations Population Division estimates that, by the year 2050, over 40 percent of the entire population of many European countries will be over age sixty. Other countries, such as Japan and Russia, are not far behind those in Europe. Many of the populations of these countries are now actually shrinking. The birth rates have dropped below replacement levels and show no sign of increasing, given current trends.[29] As economic growth improves health care in China and India and their populations survive into later life, it is expected that these countries will also face massive health-care crises.

What will huge expenditures for health care do to our federal budget, debt, and the U.S. economy? Laurence J. Kotlikoff and Scott Burns in their 2004 book, *A Coming Generational Storm*, describe what is happening in that arena. Kotlikoff is professor of economics at Boston University and a research associate at the National Bureau of Economic Research. He was senior economist for taxation and Social Security on the President's Council of Economic Advisors in the Reagan administration. Scott Burns is a writer from the *Dallas Morning News*. The book's cover has endorsements by three Nobel Prize laureates in economics: George Akerlof, professor of economics at UC Berkeley; Paul A. Samuelson, professor of economics at MIT; and James M. Buchanan, professor of economics at George Mason University.

*A Coming Generational Storm* makes some sobering points that I will briefly summarize here. By the middle of the century, we are looking at a very real $51 trillion deficit in spending. To get a sense of how much $51 trillion dollars is, consider that the total gross domestic product of the U.S. is now about $11 trillion. That means, in forty or so years, the federal debt will equal nearly five times the total economic output of the U.S. today. Where will this spending deficit come from? According to Kotlikoff, $7.2 trillion will come from Social Security's unfunded liability, and $43.1 trillion will come from Medicare expenditures. Therefore, Medicare costs make up nearly 85 percent of this deficit. Although not a Nobel Prize winner in economics, even I can predict what will happen as a $51 trillion dollar spending deficit builds. With our current debt (which increased an alarming 50 percent from $4.4 trillion to $8.5 trillion between 2000 and 2006),[30] the U.S. dollar is dropping in value compared to many foreign currencies. There is also concern about our growing trade deficit and risk of increasing inflation. These trends are likely to continue in the future, especially with the cost of the Iraq and Afghanistan wars (and future wars), homeland security, and outlays for more older adults on Medicare and Social Security.

In January 2007, Federal Reserve Chairman Ben Bernanke warned Congress that failure to take budgetary action to address the aging population will lead to serious economic harm. "Unfortunately, economic growth alone is unlikely to solve the nation's impending fiscal problems," Bernanke said. "We are experiencing what seems likely to be the calm before the storm."[31]

The problems were clear enough: increased inflation, growing deficits, decreased international credibility, and the burden of a financial deficit put on future generations. Kotlikoff, in *A Coming*

*Generational Storm*, calls his three options to address these problems "The Menu of Pain": our choices are to go bankrupt, increase taxes, and/or cut benefits (for Medicare especially). A bankrupt government that defaults on its loans to U.S. citizens and foreign countries is really not an option, so only two remain. Kotlikoff says that if, in 2003, we had increased federal income taxes by 69 percent, increased payroll taxes by 95 percent, cut federal purchases by 106 percent, or cut Social Security and Medicare by 45 percent, any one of these measures would have addressed the financial deficit. Waiting until 2008, he claimed, would increase the amounts, respectively, to 74 percent, 103 percent, 115 percent, and 47 percent.

A more reasonable solution, Kotlikoff suggested in 2003, would have been an immediate combination that raised income taxes by 17 percent and payroll taxes by 24 percent, cut federal purchases by 26 percent, and reduced Social Security and Medicare benefits by 11 percent. This plan is still a conceivable one, but as each year passes the percentages above increase. The federal government, however, is still doing nothing, and it will probably continue to do nothing in the years ahead, given powerful political forces resistant to raising taxes or cutting social or health benefits.

### Political Forces

Are there any Democrats, Republicans, or independents running for office on a platform to increase taxes or cut back Social Security and Medicare services? Americans in general are consumers, pleasure-seekers, and pain-avoiders: they are unlikely to elect anyone who pushes for these changes, now or in the future. Even the Bush administration's health-care savings accounts were turned down by Congress, and that program would have only scratched the surface of the problem.

Indeed, it will become even harder in the future to enact changes that reduce benefits. Here is the reason: according to U.S. Census projections, by 2030, nearly 40 percent of the voting population will be over age fifty-five.[32] The agenda of older adults will carry every election. Remember, these are the baby boomers, often called the "entitled" generation. This is a group that is unlikely to give up what it feels the government owes them: the Social Security and Medicare taxes that they have been paying out of their paychecks for over half a century. After all, their parents got those benefits, so why shouldn't they? So, here we go—moving toward a massive health-care crisis but ignoring all the warnings.

## HEALTH CARE SYSTEM– FAITH COMMUNITY PARTNERSHIPS

Fortunately, there are some solutions that are not entirely political and financial. One involves the role that communities might play, especially religious ones, in health care. Such solutions can be found in the very history of health care, which grew out of the religious institutions of the West.[33]

Before 372 CE, as the vast Roman Empire was beginning to crumble, there were no hospitals for care of the sick in the general population of Europe or the rest of the Western world. The first hospital was built in Caesarea (present-day Turkey) by the command of Bishop Basil. This hospital was called Basileias and was intended for the treatment of the sick, the poor, and those with leprosy. For the next one thousand years, the Church continued to build and staff hospitals throughout the Western world. Even the certification of doctors to practice medicine was a responsibility of the Church until the late middle ages, and as a result, many physicians were also monks and priests.

Until the middle of the twentieth century, most nursing care was done by religious orders in both Europe and the United States. In 1950, nearly one-quarter of all hospitalized patients in the U.S. were cared for in religious hospitals. Many hospitals today remain religiously affiliated. The bottom line is that our notion of modern health care has its roots in religious organizations. That influence continues to be felt, and it remains a major resource for the crisis of the twenty-first century.

Religious organizations will not be isolated from the coming crisis. They will feel the health care brunt as much as the federal government. Many older adults will be members of faith groups (as almost two-thirds of Americans are today). Thus, religious organizations will have more older members struggling with chronic health problems. Many of the younger members will have parents and grandparents who need care at home, since few other options will exist.

No doubt, health ministries in religious communities will become more frequent and relied on in the decades ahead. A parish or congregational nurse (a registered nurse who is a member of the congregation) will often lead such health ministries and will be responsible for organizing and training volunteers to carry out health programs.[34] The first responsibility of such ministries will be to promote healthy lifestyles, diet, and exercise among members, as well as to conduct disease screening (blood pressure, blood sugar, and cholesterol checks). The aim will be to keep members of the congregation healthy so that they will be the givers of support to others, rather than the consumers of health care. As more and more older adults need to be cared for in the community, healthy older and younger volunteers from faith communities could begin to assist the growing number of sick elders who would otherwise fall through the widening cracks in the government-funded health-care system.

Other health professionals besides parish nurses could also play an important supportive role in this endeavor. Physicians could assist the parish nurse in educating members of the congregation about maintaining health, as well as on detecting and managing disease. Health-care funders (including Medicare and private insurance companies) could be called upon to help support the salaries of parish nurses, something that would enable them to spend more of their time doing this work. Keeping people at home and out of the hospital will help save the health-care system huge amounts of money.

Because the pressure of diminishing financial resources and increasing health-care needs is not yet high enough, this model of collaborative partnerships between health-care systems and religious communities is more the exception than the rule today. Nevertheless, in places like Florida and certain areas of the Midwest, these collaborations are beginning to appear. The Seventh-day Adventist, Lutheran Advocate Health Care, and Catholic Ascension Health Care systems have been particularly active in this regard. The same is true for Mennonite and Brethren health-care systems. The Adventist's Florida Hospital has been exemplary in initiating partnerships with faith communities throughout Florida to help meet the health-care needs of older adults.[35] There is little doubt in my mind that that future economic pressures will force faith communities and health-care systems to confront this common crisis together. For these partnerships to work most effectively, however, they must be developed now while there is still some breathing room, not in forty years when the need is urgent and circumstances are out of control.[36]

## CONCLUSIONS

The latter part of the twentieth century saw a rapid rise in research examining the relationships between religion, spirituality, and health, and that trend has continued into the first decade of the current century. The research is now of much higher quality than earlier, when such investigations had little funding or institutional support. There are many plausible reasons why health-care professionals should address a patient's spiritual needs, backed by the research described above. In the past fifteen years, nearly 70 percent of U.S. medical schools have begun to offer courses on religion, spirituality, and medicine. The majority of these are required for all medical students. But the question remains: can this new under-standing by health professionals and an increasing role played by religious groups meet the economic and political crisis that will likely soon transform health care? While persuading voters to make sacrifices may be impossible, a new movement of religious commu-nity–health care partnerships could provide an important safety valve, building on a historic precedent that has been operating for nearly two thousand years.

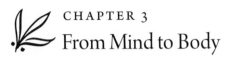

CHAPTER 3

# From Mind to Body

HAVE YOU NOTICED that you are more susceptible to colds when going through a time of unusually high stress—perhaps related to problems at work or in school, or when dealing with grief over the death of a loved one or the loss of an important relationship? It is common knowledge that, when people get angry and upset over mishaps or injustices, their faces turn red, their hearts race, and perhaps they suffer a headache. Their blood pressure goes up as well. When you are anxious or scared, you have surely noticed how your mouth gets dry. You may even have to run to the bathroom a bit more often than usual. These are all physiological reactions to stress, and that is what this chapter is about—the effects of stress on the body.

The influence that emotions have on the natural healing systems in the body is an important area of research if we want to understand the ways that religious or spiritual factors can affect health. When talking about religion, we cannot discount that supernatural mechanisms may be involved. But from the viewpoint of science— the approach of this book—the supernatural is something that can neither be proved nor disproved. Scientific research is only capable of looking at natural explanations. Therefore, the most obvious and plausible "natural" way that religion might impact physical health is through pathways that are psychological, social, and behavioral. Studies of the effects of psychological and social factors on the physical body over the past two and a half decades have resulted in the emergence of an entirely new scientific field of research called psychoneuroimmunology.

In this chapter, I review research published in mainstream medical, psychology, and public-health science journals demonstrating how psychological and social factors can influence physical health. If we can establish such pathways, then this may help to explain how religion (a powerful psychological and social factor) could influence health.

## PSYCHOLOGICAL FACTORS AND HEALTH

A growing body of research suggests that psychological factors, particularly negative emotions—stress, anxiety, depression, burnout, anger, and hostility—can adversely affect physiological systems, susceptibility to disease, and medical outcomes. In his seminal article on allostatic load, published in the *New England Journal of Medicine*, Bruce McEwen examined how psychological factors could influence physical health through the hypothalamic-pituitary-adrenal axis, the autonomic nervous system, the metabolic system, and the cardiovascular and the immune systems.[1] These are all body functions that help people adapt physically to everyday life. With this larger picture in mind, let's look at some of the physiological processes that take place when a person experiences psychological or social stress.

### Immune Function
In both human and animal studies, depression and other forms of psychological stress have been associated with impaired natural killer (NK) cell activity, cytotoxic T-cell functions, and increased levels of cytokines such as interleukin-6.[2] Stress has been shown to influence immune responses to vaccinations for influenza virus, pneumococcal bacterium, meningococcal bacterium, and hepatitis B virus.[3] Furthermore, stress-reducing therapies may facilitate a more vigorous response by the body to vaccines against viruses

and bacteria.[4] Psychosocial interventions have also been shown to have a positive impact on a number of other immune parameters, including lymphoproliferative responses to mitogens and level of circulating white blood cells.[5] Particularly notable is that persons who score high on a "sense of coherence" (i.e., people who perceive life events as meaningful and capable of being mastered versus as threats) may be partially protected from such stress-induced immune changes.[6]

### Endocrine Function

Numerous studies have demonstrated that negative emotions such as depression can influence hormone levels in the body, especially cortisol and catecholamine levels.[7] These hormones are known to suppress immune functions.[8] For example, studies have shown that increases in serum cortisol can impair immune functions sufficiently to allow the reactivation of latent viruses such as the Epstein-Barr virus that is responsible for mononucleosis.[9] Cortisol has also been shown to enhance cancer growth in animal models, especially in older animals.[10] Catecholamines, such as epinephrine and norepinephrine, are likewise influenced by negative emotions or negative events, and these hormones are known to directly or indirectly affect immune function.[11] For example, catecholamines released during psychological stress have been shown to suppress NK cell activity, macrophage activity, $T_H$ production of IL-12, tumor necrosis factor, and other inflammatory factors necessary for a healthy immune response.[12]

### Cytokine Production

Cytokines are blood proteins that regulate the body's immune response to infection and injury. Cytokines such as interleukin-6 (IL-6) both promote inflammation and stimulate the production of cortisol, which then reduces immune responses to control inflammatory responses, all part of a carefully regulated negative feedback loop (to keep the body from over-responding to infections or injury). Studies have shown that depression and psychosocial stress lead to elevated levels of cytokines such as IL-6.[13] A high level of IL-6 is typical in patients who have weakened immune systems from HIV infection or as a result of having AIDS and is also common in patients with age-related immune-system cancers such as non-Hodgkin's lymphoma or chronic lymphocytic leukemia, reflecting a decline in healthy immune function with age.[14]

## Metabolic Disorders

Psychological stress and negative emotions have been associated with a number of adverse metabolic states. These include the development of insulin resistance. For example, Raikkonen and colleagues found that feelings of excessive tiredness, lack of energy, increased irritability, demoralization, and hostility were associated with the development of insulin resistance (a major risk factor for Type II diabetes).[15] Similarly, Zhang and colleagues more recently reported that persons who scored high on both psychological stress and hostility were at increased risk for insulin resistance.[16] Most recently, Melamed and colleagues examined 633 persons over a three to five-year period, finding that those with negative emotions had over an 80 percent increased likelihood of developing Type II diabetes, an effect that persisted after controlling for numerous other risk factors.[17]

## Neurological Disease

Chronic stress in both animal and human studies has been shown to decrease neurogenesis (nerve growth) in the hippocampal region of the brain (the memory center).[18] For example, Wilson and colleagues recently followed one thousand older Catholic clergy to examine the effects of chronic stress on cognitive impairment/dementia.[19] During follow-up, 326 persons died (mean age eighty-five) and 219 underwent brain autopsy. Results indicated that chronic stress was associated with a higher likelihood of dementia and a lower level of cognition prior to death.

### Cardiovascular Disease

Psychological factors such as stress and depression can increase the risk of cardiovascular disease or worsen its course. No other area of research in psychosomatic medicine is growing more rapidly. Here I examine associations with coronary artery disease, congestive heart failure, hypertension, and stroke.

**Coronary Artery Disease.** Coronary Artery Disease (CAD) has been linked with depression, chronic stress, and anger/hostility in numerous studies. For example, in a sample of 1,551 adults who were initially free of heart disease, Pratt and colleagues found that a diagnosis of major depression predicted a 4.5-fold increased risk of myocardial infarction and that a history of chronic milder depression predicted a 2.7-fold increased risk.[20] One of the most impressive studies on depression and CAD was by Blumenthal and colleagues who followed 817 patients undergoing coronary artery bypass grafting for up to twelve years.[21] After carefully controlling for traditional risk factors, patients with moderate to severe depression at baseline had a 2.4-fold increased risk of mortality.

*Chronic* stress can also affect CAD mortality. One study of stressed caregivers followed for four years found that they had a 63 percent greater mortality than noncaregiver controls.[22] In another study, women caring for a sick spouse for nine hours per day or more had twice the risk of CAD morbidity over four years as other women.[23] Even women caring for healthy children may be at increased risk of CAD. A study of women who cared for non-ill children more than twenty-one hours per week or grandchildren more than nine hours per week were shown to be at increased risk for CAD morbidity compared to women without such responsibilities.[24]

Hostility has been shown to be a robust predictor of cardiovascular disease and cardiovascular mortality over many decades. Although the Type A personality has long been known to increase CAD, a review of this literature concluded that the hostility component of Type A personality is the primary factor explaining the increased CAD.[25] For example, one study found that men with high levels of anger (upper 20 percent) experienced 2.5 times more non-fatal heart attacks, fatal CAD, and angina pectoris than those in the lowest 20 percent during seven years of follow-up.[26] Hostility has even been shown to predict the development of coronary artery calcification over time, as investigators found in a study of 374 healthy adults ages eighteen to thirty followed over ten years.[27]

**Congestive Heart Failure.** Depression adversely affects the course of illness in patients with congestive heart failure, the heart condition that often results from years of CAD-caused myocardial ischemia. For example, Jiang and colleagues followed 374 patients with congestive hearth failure over one year, examining the effects of baseline depression (14 percent with major depression) on mortality.[28] Major depression increased the risk of mortality 2.5-fold at three months and 2.2-fold at one year. Furthermore, the presence of depression nearly doubled the risk of hospital readmission by three months and over tripled the risk by one year. These effects were adjusted for age, New York Heart Association functional class, baseline ejection fraction, and cause of congestive heart failure. Likewise, Sullivan and colleagues followed 142 outpatients with advanced congestive heart failure over an average of three years, assessing the effects of baseline depression on cardiac outcomes.[29] A total of 29 percent of subjects were diagnosed with depressive disorder at the beginning of the study. These patients were two and one-half times more likely to die or require heart transplantation. Adjusting for other social, demographic, and cardiac predictors did not substantially alter this finding. In addition, depressed patients had significantly more hospitalizations and clinic visits during the first year of observation.

**Hypertension.** Psychological stress is known to affect blood pressure and increase the risk of hypertension. For example, Ming and colleagues followed 218 men over twenty years with either no blood-

tionship between cortisol and
stress and low social support
els, an indicator of poorer dia-

n association between age-
upport. For example, Van
lationship of marital status
itive decline over ten years
in Finland, Italy, and the
ducation, country, smok-
ine cognition, investiga-
ho were unmarried, who
perienced twice the rate
ied or living with some-

d as a cause of cognitive
ted or have low social
, Sapolsky has hypoth-
e memory cells in the
ay simulate sufficient
rophy and adversely

ties or social isola-
in numerous stud-
tality in a number
nd Marmot for a
t studies confirm
colleagues exam-
her mortality for
was almost two

ychological stress or neg-

out these links between
and cardiovascular func-
stion, remember the role
social support and social

mmune function and lone-
ships, social support, and
edical students, feelings of
K cell activity, higher uri-
eripheral blood leukocytes
rm close, intimate relation-
unity. For example, in one
ts of attachment style on
ere interested in the effects
s defined as difficulty trust-
omfortable with emotional
partner for support. In that
achment-related avoidance
Perceived Stress Scale) pre-

ciated with social factors in
xample, social isolation and
al models have been associ-
altered autonomic nervous
have reported similar results.
and women, assessing social
alivary cortisol every three
tional and longitudinal anal-

pressure elevation or only mild blood-pressure elevation.[30] All men were involved in a high-stress occupation (air-traffic controllers). Those with increased cardiovascular reactivity to psychological stress at baseline had an increase in long-term risk of hypertension. Findings are similar for depression. Davidson and colleagues found that symptoms of depression predicted the early development of hypertension in a sample of 3,343 young adults, especially for African Americans in the sample.[31] High depression scores predicted a 2.8-fold increased risk of developing hypertension during a five-year follow-up in African American subjects.

Hostility has also been shown to significantly increase the risk of developing long-term hypertension. In a sample of 3,308 persons ages eighteen to thirty, the risk of hypertension at fifteen-year follow-up for those in the highest hostility quartile was 84 percent higher compared to those in the lowest hostility quartile.[32]

**Stroke.** Since high blood pressure is a strong predictor of stroke, it is not surprising that a number of studies have found that negative emotions such as depression or chronic stress can increase the risk of stroke and affect stroke mortality rates. For example, an eighteen-year follow-up of 11,216 men initially without evidence of cardiovascular disease found that subjects depressed at baseline were twice as likely to die from stroke after adjusting for a large number of other risk factors.[33] Likewise, Lewis and colleagues examined negative attitudes and mental adjustment as predictors of stroke and stroke survival in 372 patients followed for three to five years.[34] In that study, fatalism and helplessness/hopelessness were both associated with decreased survival after adjusting for other relevant factors. Having a diagnosis of bipolar disorder has also been associated with a greater risk of stroke in at least one recent report.[35]

**Infection.** Studies show that psychological stress can alter susceptibility to respiratory viruses such as the common cold.[36] Likewise, more persons develop cold symptoms after infection with

respiratory viruses if stressful life events have [
Distressed anxious persons also have a dela[
shorter-lived immune response, which is associa[
susceptibility to cold viruses and longer-lastin[
noted above, stressed individuals do not develop[
immune response to vaccination, and a poorer resp[
predicts increased rates of infection.[39]

**Wound Healing.** The immune system plays a vital ro[
of wounds due to injury or surgical operation.[40] Stud[
mals and humans document that stress can adversely[
healing, in part due to stress-induced increases in serur[
changes in immune function. This has been shown in [
and in numerous studies of stressed humans—whether[
dents during exam week, middle-aged couples experienc[
marital interactions, patients undergoing elective surg[
sons caring for a loved ones with Alzheimer's disease.[41] Pl[
may also impair immune function and interfere with wou[
through similar mechanisms.[42] Psychological distress inc[
risk of bacterial infection in a wound after injury, which ma[
ute to slower wound healing during stressful life periods.[43]

**Cancer.** Although the evidence linking negative psych[
states and stress to cancer is weaker than it is for the link b[
stress and cardiovascular disease, negative emotions in[
studies predict an increased prevalence of cancer or prec[
ous lesions. This may be particularly true for persons who e[
ence chronic negative psychological states such as depressio[
example, Brown and colleagues examined relationships bet[
depressive symptoms and survival time (up to ten years) an[
205 cancer patients.[44] Depressive symptoms were the most col[
tent psychological predictor of shortened survival time, indep[
dent of several known demographic and medical risk factors. Th[
is also evidence of an increased prevalence of lymphatic and hen[

---

ence physiological systems sensitive to ps[
ative emotions.

What, then, is the research saying al[
social factors and immune, endocrine, [
tions in the body? As we turn to this qu[
that religious involvement plays in the [
networks of many people.

### Immune Function

Research has identified links between in[
liness, ability to form intimate relation[
social network size. Even in healthy me[
loneliness have been linked to lower N[
nary cortisol, and reduced response of p[
to phytohemagglutinin.[49] Inability to fo[
ships may also negatively impact imm[
study researchers examined the effec[
immune function. In particular, they w[
of attachment-related avoidance. This i[
ing or depending on others, feeling unc[
closeness, and being reluctant to ask a[
study of sixty-one healthy nurses, att[
and perceived stress (measured by the[
dicted lower NK cell cytotoxicity.[50]

### Endocrine and Metabolic Function

Stress hormone levels have been asso[
both animal and human studies. For [
chronic social stress in primate anim[
ated with high levels of cortisol and [
system activity.[51] Studies in humans [
Rosal and colleagues studied 146 men[
support, psychological stress, and [
months for one year.[52] Both cross-se[

---

For example, prior to male [
sitting activities, there is a [
in cortisol levels.[78] Other st[
and caring behaviors invol[
changes in prolactin and ot[
sequences for immune and [

Although research in hu[
report physical changes i[
ing in other helping behav[
*Homes and Gardens*, an ar[
Readers were asked to w[
helping experiences mad[
study, the results were i[
246 respondents indica[
when helping others. A[
percent felt stronger ar[
percent felt less depres[
worth.

There is some evid[
ity to stimulate feelin[
reported by these re[
have hypothesized t[
blood vessels near t[
"warmth" in the bo[
ther research is ne[
involved in prosoc[

## CONCLUSION

From this sample[
it is clear that p[
and social relati[
physical health.[
to have negativ[

ious and fearful. How did they cope? According to a study published during the week following those attacks, 90 percent of Americans turned to religion for comfort and support.[2] In some areas of the United States, nearly one-half of hospitalized patients indicate that their religious beliefs and practices are *the most important way* that they cope with illness and life changes caused by illness.

Let's probe this strategy for coping with illness more closely. One study looked at 330 patients consecutively admitted to the medical, neurological, and cardiology services of a large academic teaching hospital. Researchers found that 42 percent of them reported— spontaneously and without prompting—that religious beliefs and practices were the primary factor that enabled them to cope.[3] When asked to rate the extent to which religion was used in coping on a scale of one to ten, 40 percent indicated ten, and 50 percent indicated somewhere between five and ten (where five indicated a moderate extent and ten, the most important factor that kept them going). Only 10 percent of subjects rated anything below five. A second study of 838 consecutively hospitalized patients over age fifty found that 98 percent were affiliated with a religious group, 38 percent attended religious services weekly (despite health problems), 81 percent prayed privately once a day or more, and 51 percent read the Bible or other inspirational literature at least several times each week.[4]

Both of these aforementioned studies were done in North Carolina, but they reflect national trends as well. A survey of 382 randomly selected persons in California asked what kinds of unconventional remedies were used to deal with musculoskeletal pain complaints.[5] Prayer was the most common of all remedies mentioned (44 percent). Prayer was also ranked the second most helpful in a long list of other unconventional therapies for pain; 54 percent of those who used prayer said it was "very helpful." In another study of 406 patients with chronic mental illness, conducted at a Los Angeles County mental health facility, more than 80 percent indicated they used religion to cope.[6] The majority of these patients spent nearly half of their total coping time in religious activities such as prayer. The authors concluded that religious coping was a "pervasive and potentially effective method of coping for persons with mental illness, thus warranting its integration into psychiatric and psychological practice."

Religious coping is also prevalent in countries outside the United States. Rammohan and colleagues surveyed sixty Hindu caregivers of schizophrenic patients in India, finding that 97 percent believed in God, 58 percent considered their religious beliefs an integral part of life, and 50 percent viewed religion as a source of solace, strength, and guidance.[7] Another study compared cancer patients in Switzerland and Egypt on how they coped with illness.[8] In this comparison, Kesselring and colleagues found that, while 38 percent of Swiss patients indicated that faith in God and prayer were important sources of support, 92 percent of Egyptian patients (Muslim) indicated the same. Similarly, a study of seventy-nine psychiatric patients at Broken Hill Base Hospital in New South Wales, found that 79 percent rated spirituality as very important, 82 percent thought their therapist should be aware of their spiritual beliefs and needs, and 67 percent indicated that their spirituality helped them to cope with psychological pain.[9] Thus, if religious beliefs and practices such as prayer help people to cope and reduce stress level, then such activities should also be related to physical health, given what we know about the effects of psychological stress and depression on the body.

## SOURCE OF SOCIAL SUPPORT

In almost every study to date, religious involvement has been related to both the amount of social support and the quality of that support. In an earlier review of this research, nineteen of twenty quantitative studies found significant positive relationships.[10] This is especially true in older adults. For example, Cutler found that older adults are more likely to be members of religious organizations than of any other social groups, and church membership was the only type of social involvement that predicted greater life satisfaction and happiness (after controlling for other factors).[11] Likewise, in a survey of 4,522 randomly sampled persons in northern Alabama, among all variables measured, informal interpersonal contact was the strongest predictor of life satisfaction. This was true, however, only if friendships were church-based. Furthermore, for older African Americans in that study, greater life satisfaction was due almost entirely to greater contact with church friends. Not only is religious involvement associated with higher social support, the health effects of church-related support appear to be greater than the effects of support obtained outside of the church.[12] Recent research confirms these reports.[13]

This is especially true for persons with health problems whom health professionals are likely to encounter in medical settings. My colleagues and I found that, for a majority of older medical patients, 80 percent or more of their closest friends came from their religious congregations.[14] Religious support may be particularly durable during times of medical illness, when people are less able to hold up their part of the social contract. Social support from religious sources is motivated by more than just the social contract that secular sources of support are based on. Religious persons provide support to others not only because they want to but because "loving thy neighbor" and caring for the needy are part of the religious belief system itself. It is *especially* when the other is in need and unable to return social favors that people of faith are called to care for one another. The belief is that God will reward them for such altruistic actions, either in this life or the next. Thus, the social support they provide persists long after the other person is unable to return the support.

## BEHAVIORAL MODIFIER

The daily, habitual decisions that we make in response to life's temptations and challenges are often influenced by religious beliefs. This is particularly true when such decisions have ethical implications and potentially stressful consequences. Here are some examples:

: Should I cheat a little on my taxes? If I cheat and get caught, then financial stress (or even imprisonment) could result; if I cheat and don't get caught, then I'll probably do it again and again, until I do get caught.

: Should I speed while driving or otherwise act irresponsibly? The consequence could be an auto accident that leaves another person or even myself disabled for life.

: Should I expose myself to pornography in magazines or movies or on the Internet? If I do, this could affect my future sex life in unintended ways that could hurt others and me.

: Should I cheat a little in my marriage? If I do, then marital stress or divorce could be the consequence.

: Should I spend time with my family or go golfing with my friends? Long-term family relationships may suffer, and this could lead to lack of support or even abandonment later in life when I really need those relationships.

: Should I help out my associate at work faced with a difficult situation even if I'm not likely to benefit? Failure to do so will probably mean that my colleague will not help me out of a jam when I need help, and it may even affect how my other colleagues view me.

: As a teenager, should I have sexual relations before marriage? If so, then I could get pregnant or become a father, affecting my education and career plans, or I could develop a venereal disease that may recur later.

: Should I use drugs, smoke cigarettes, or drink alcohol when my stress level gets high? If I do, I could get addicted, or could be arrested for driving under the influence.

These are just a few examples of decisions that confront us every day, choices that religious beliefs may influence. The consequences of such decisions could have a major impact on our emotional well-being and social and work relationships, which, in turn, could influence our physical health. Religious training in a family, school, or church setting during youth helps to instill honesty, dependability, purity, responsibility, concern for others that can influence future decisions throughout life.

For example, Wallace and Forman analyzed data from a random sample of five thousand high school students as part of the Monitoring the Future Project conducted by the University of Michigan.[15] Religious importance was inversely related to carrying a weapon to school, interpersonal violence, driving while drinking, riding while drinking, failure to wear seat belts, binge drinking, marijuana use, poor-quality diet, lack of exercise, and poor sleep. Frequency of religious attendance was also inversely related to injury behaviors, substance use, and many risky lifestyle behaviors. Other studies conducted both prior to and since the Wallace and Forman study support these findings in youth and adulthood, as the research reviewed below documents.

*Crime and Delinquency*

In the *Handbook of Religion and Health*, my colleagues and I identify thirty-six studies prior to the year 2000 that examined the relationship between religious involvement and criminal behavior.[16] Nearly 80 percent of these studies reported significantly lower rates of delinquency or criminal behavior among those who were more religious. For example, analyzing data from a national random sample of 11,995 high school seniors, Stark found that those who attended religious services regularly were significantly less likely to be involved in delinquent or criminal behavior.[17] Since the year 2000, other research has replicated these findings. Johnson surveyed 2,300 black males ages sixteen to twenty-four from Boston, Chicago, or Philadelphia, finding that religious involvement was inversely associated with drug-related and nondrug-related crimes.[18] In another study, this research group reported that prison inmates who completed a faith-based prison program involving prayer and scripture study were only about half as likely to be arrested or reincarcerated during a two-year follow-up, compared to a matched control group of other prisoners.[19]

Physically abused youth at high risk for future criminal involvement may also be protected to some degree from such adverse consequences if they are more involved in a religious community.[20] Amount of time spent with a chaplain also predicted positive outcomes in delinquent youth in a residential treatment program.[21] In the latter study, time spent with a chaplain was significantly correlated with completion of the residential treatment program, stable living situation at twelve months after discharge, and cost of care, all in positive directions. Finally, Butts and colleagues' review of this literature indicated a consistent inverse relationship between religious involvement and crime.[22]

### Alcohol Use

A 2001 press release from the National Center on Addiction and Substance Abuse (CASA) at Columbia University reported results on the relationship between religion and substance abuse from the analysis of three national datasets (National Household Survey, CASA's National Survey of American Attitudes on Substance Abuse, and the General Social Survey).[23] Adults who do not consider religious beliefs to be important were more than three times likelier to binge drink (versus those whose religious beliefs were very important), and those who never attended religious services were almost seven times more likely to drink than those who attended weekly or more. Similarly, teens who said that religion was not important were nearly three times more likely to drink or binge drink, and those who never attended religious services were twice as likely to drink, compared to weekly attendees.

This report is consistent with a review of the research prior to the year 2000. Of eighty-six studies on the religiosity–alcohol relationship, seventy-six found that greater religiousness was associated with less alcohol intake, alcohol abuse, and alcohol dependence.[24] More recent studies confirm these earlier reports.[25] Religious or spiritual involvement may be particularly important for recovery among minority groups, such as Native Americans, Hispanics, and African Americans.[26]

## Drug Use

As with alcohol, religious involvement is inversely correlated with illicit drug use, and many of these studies concentrate on younger adults. An earlier review of religious involvement and drug use found that, of fifty-two studies conducted before the year 2000, forty-eight reported significant inverse relationships between religious activity and drug use.[27] More recent longitudinal research reports similar findings. For example, in a study of 501 adolescents ages fourteen to nineteen attending eighteen high schools across southern California, Sussman and colleagues found that, after controlling for baseline drug use, spirituality predicted significantly less marijuana and stimulant use at one-year follow-up.[28] Likewise, White and colleagues examined how protective factors in late adolescence predicted substance use after high school and during the first year of college in a sample of 319 students. Students were interviewed on graduating from high school and again six months later. Results indicated that having fewer substance-abusing friends and higher religiosity protected against future use of marijuana and other substances.[29]

As with alcohol, religion has been reported to be particularly important as a protective factor against drug abuse for members of minority communities. Steinman and Zimmerman prospectively interviewed 705 African American youths annually throughout high school, assessing religious activity and cigarette and marijuana use.[30] The results of growth-curve analyses indicated a negative association between religious activity and substance-abuse behaviors. Higher levels of religious activity in ninth grade predicted smaller increases in marijuana use among males and less cigarette use among females. Likewise, in a four-year prospective study of 318 African American high school dropouts, Kogan and colleagues found that religious involvement predicted conventional peer affiliations and positive life orientation, which were the major factors that influenced later substance abuse in these youth.[31] Substance-abuse programs in African American faith communities hold particular promise for stemming the tide of drug and alcohol abuse among young blacks.[32] Recently, mainstream alcohol and drug-abuse experts have emphasized the role that spirituality can play in facilitating recovery or prevention and have outlined a research agenda focused on measurement, longitudinal study, and involvement of faith communities in facilitating behavioral change.[33]

## Divorce

In a review of studies prior to the year 2000 examining relationships between religious involvement and marital stability, thirty-five of thirty-eight quantitative studies found greater marital happiness or stability among those couples who were either more religious or had similar religious backgrounds.[34] More recent research continues to show strong associations between religious involvement, religious homogamy (same religious denomination for husband and wife), marital quality, and stability.[35] For example, a national random survey of 4,999 women ages twenty-five to thirty-four years conducted between 1974 and 2002 involving the General Social Survey found that frequency of religious attendance and degree of religious fundamentalism both predicted positive responses to the statement, "Divorce should be more difficult to obtain." Religious attendance and fundamentalism were among the strongest predictors of this attitude among dozens of other characteristics.[36]

Studies in Middle Eastern countries report similar findings. For example, Hunler and Gencoz surveyed 184 persons (ninety-two couples) living in Turkey.[37] After controlling for other factors, including duration of marriage, marital style, educational level, mental health, and submissive acts, researchers found in this largely Muslim sample that great religiousness predicted greater marital satisfaction.

Mullins and colleagues found that a higher concentration of religious affiliation in a county predicted a lower divorce rate, after controlling for fifteen other covariates.[38] Concentration of affiliation ranked ninth in predictive strength among fifteen other characteristics and was more influential than the age category fifteen to thirty-four years, ethnicity, employment in manufacturing occupations, or residence in the Northeast. In their latest report, Mullins and colleagues examined the effects of specific religious affiliation concentrations (again based on analyses at the county level) on divorce rate.[39] They found that, contrary to expectation, affiliation with conservative Protestant churches (Southern Baptist, Assemblies of God, Church of God, Evangelical, Holiness, Pentecostal, etc.) was associated with the highest divorce rate compared to counties with higher affiliations with miscellaneous Protestant (Mennonite, Amish, Quakers, Brethren, etc.), moderate Protestant (American Baptists, Disciples of Christ, Lutheran, United Methodist), Mormon, and Catholic affiliations, in that order, after controlling for other covariates, including income, employment status, type of occupation, ethnicity, gender, region of the United States, urban versus rural, age group, and other variables.

## Sexual Promiscuity

The impact that religious teachings have on sexual behaviors is evident from published research, despite the stories that appear almost daily in the headlines of newspapers about the sexual misconduct of clergy. A review of research published before the year 2000 found that thirty-eight studies had examined the relationship between religion and sexual attitudes or behaviors. Of those, thirty-seven (97 percent) found that persons who were more religiously involved reported lower rates or more negative attitudes toward nonmarital sexual relations than less religious subjects.[40] What is particularly notable is that most of these studies (thirty-two of thirty-eight) were conducted among young persons (i.e., adolescents or college students). Such attitudes during youth may influence sexual behaviors throughout life.

More recent research in both the United States and other countries supports these findings, stressing the importance of religious commitment, authority-related conformity, peer-group religiosity, and religion's relationship to adolescent adjustment.[41] Religious involvement may be particularly important for reducing high-risk sexual activities.[42] Other research suggests that religious activity, particularly frequent attendance at religious services, has a strong delaying effect on the timing of first intercourse, although its ability to influence adolescent sexual behavior may weaken after first sex actually occurs. Furthermore, greater personal conservatism increases the likelihood of having unprotected sex.[43]

These findings on religion and sexual promiscuity are particularly strong in women and may be due to religion's prescribing different sex-related norms, such as the importance of virginity before marriage, and influencing norms and sanctions that regulate sexual risk-taking and other risk behaviors.[44] Religious teachings encourage people to have sexual relations only within the marital relationship, not before marriage, not while married with other partners, and not after marriage following divorce or widowhood, unless remarriage takes place. These teachings may not mesh well with current cultural values, but they could have a wide range of consequences, in terms of marital stability, satisfaction, and trust, and in terms of risk of contracting HIV/AIDS, herpes, syphilis, gonorrhea, and other venereal diseases.

### Venereal Disease

Early studies reported that sexually transmitted diseases such as trichomoniasis were less frequent among religiously active women.[45] The dramatic drop in HIV/AIDS in certain countries of Africa, the East, and the Caribbean islands has been attributed in part to the reduction in number of sexual partners.[46] In study after study, religious involvement has been associated with fewer sexual partners for women, men, and college students.[47] There is also evidence that the prevalence of HIV/AIDS is less common among members of religions such as Islam that strongly advocate single-partner sexual relationships within marriage.[48] Strong parental disapproval of sexual activity during adolescence may be a key mediator between religious involvement and risk of developing sexually transmitted diseases.[49] The greater likelihood of religious adolescents having unprotected sex, however, may partially neutralize the health effects of religion on reducing promiscuity.

In summary, there is little doubt that the constraining influence of religious teachings and personal religious commitment can help to reduce behaviors that lead to greater physical disease and adversely affect health outcomes. The fact that many of these influences are first felt during childhood, adolescence, and young adulthood underscores their potential to continue to impact health throughout adulthood. Some critics have dismissed religion's effects by claiming that they can all be explained simply on the basis of healthy lifestyles. This critique, however, is misguided. The notion that religion's effects on health can partially be explained by healthy lifestyles in no way minimizes the powerful contribution that religion makes to health and wellness, but rather helps to explain how it does so.

## PROSOCIAL AGENT

Prosocial activities, such as acts of altruism and volunteering, are also related to religious involvement, and most religions encourage other-helping activities. Because of relationships between such activities and both mental and physical health, this may further help to explain how religion impacts health.

One thing is certain: the research is unambiguous in finding that religious involvement lies behind much of the altruistic behavior that occurs in the United States and around the world. For example, 70 percent of all volunteering among older adults is done within a religious setting, and those who attend religious services most often are also most likely to volunteer.[50] In one study of over seventeen hundred persons, the strongest predictors of volunteering were religiosity, religious identity, religious socialization, extent of religious social networks, and, especially, level of involvement in church activities.[51]

The Independent Sector is a nonprofit organization that helps support charities, foundations, and corporate-giving programs in the United States and around the world.[52] Based on a 2001 national U.S. survey of four thousand adults by the Independent Sector, volunteers were more likely than nonvolunteers to belong to a religious organization (76 percent versus 58 percent, respectively).[53] Researchers also found that people who attended religious services at least once a month gave more than twice as much annually to charities as those who attended less frequently or not at all ($2,151 versus $867, respectively). In fact, regular church attendees account for 80 percent of all charitable giving. Based on percentage of income, weekly attendees give 2.8 percent of their incomes, while those attending less than weekly give 1.6 percent, and nonattendees give 1.1 percent.[54]

Schwartz and colleagues examined the relationship between altruistic activities, such as helping others, with mental and physical health in a random national sample of 2,016 members of the Presbyterian Church.[55] Helping others was significantly correlated with better mental health, even after controlling for age, gender, stressful life events, income, general health, and religious characteristics. Predictors of giving help included increased prayer activities, satisfaction with prayer life, positive religious coping, and being a church elder.

Experimental studies have also demonstrated that religion-motivated acts of altruism are neither simply a result of moral hypocrisy nor reflect self-delusion, as some have claimed.[56] Saroglou and colleagues conducted four experimental studies involving hypothetical scenarios to examine the role of religion in altruism.[57] In the first study of 106 subjects, those who were more religious tended to use less aggression when dealing with daily hassles. In the second study, religiosity among a sample of 105 female studies was correlated with willingness to help others. In the third and fourth studies, involving 315 and 274 subjects, respectively, religious persons not only reported higher altruistic behavior and empathy but were also judged that way more often by their peers. The investigators concluded that the altruistic behavior of religious persons in these studies was not due simply to gender, social desirability, security of attachment, degree of empathy, or level of honesty.

## Conclusions

People frequently depend on religious beliefs and practices to cope with stressful life circumstances, loss of loved ones, and loss of health and independence, and often say that these beliefs and practices give them a sense of control and help them to adapt more quickly to difficult circumstances. Religion is also an important source of social support, especially for older adults, minorities, and those with health problems.

Furthermore, religious beliefs and teachings encourage people to make better decisions that help to decrease the likelihood of being in highly stressful situations (imprisoned, divorced, unhappily married). These beliefs may often reduce negative health behaviors, such as excessive alcohol use, illicit drug use, cigarette smoking, and sexual promiscuity. Finally, religious involvement increases the likelihood that persons will be generous with their time (volunteering) and finances in helping others and becoming involved in altruistic, prosocial kinds of activities. This research builds on what we already know about psychological and social pathways to better health.

Thus far, I have tried to show how psychological, social, and behavioral factors can influence health. I have also examined how religious involvement may influence physical health through each of these pathways. In the next section of the book, I will look at relationships between religion/spirituality and more specific areas of health, beginning first with emotional or mental health.

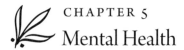

## CHAPTER 5
# Mental Health

As we are told by the family of Mrs. Harris, she died peacefully. She even had a little smile on her face, the same facial expression her friends and family had seen whenever she was deeply content. How did Mrs. Harris do it? More specifically, what role did her faith play in helping her to stay calm and peaceful during health and illness, during good times and bad, even when she was dying? Here I discuss research that has tried to better understand the relationship between faith and mental health. My definition of mental health is simple: it is the absence of mental disorder (depression, suicide, anxiety) and the presence of positive emotions (well-being, optimism, hope). As we saw in chapter 3, mental health may have a direct impact on physical health.

## Depression

Everyone perhaps experiences it to some degree, or at some moment—depression. In its fullest form, however, depression is a psychological condition associated with loss of appetite (or excessive appetite), loss of energy, difficulty concentrating, difficulty sleeping, feeling restless (or moving more slowly), loss of interest or lack of motivation, feeling sad or irritable, feeling worthless or excessively guilty, and so trapped in these painful feelings that suicide may be considered the only way out. To be called a depressive disorder, this psychological condition must interfere with a person's ability to function at work, in social relationships, or in recreational activities. A true depressive disorder is a serious mental condition that carries a 15 percent lifetime risk of dying from suicide.[1]

Depression is especially common among patients seen in medical settings, such as acute-care hospitals and nursing homes. In acute-care hospitals, as many as one out of every two patients fulfill criteria for a depressive disorder.[2] Depression rates are likewise high in long-term care settings among patients, especially among those who are not cognitively impaired or demented.[3] Depression, in turn, affects motivation toward recovery and is associated with longer hospital stays and poorer medical outcomes, including an increased mortality risk from medical causes other than suicide (see chapter 3).[4]

There is a consistent and replicable inverse relationship between religious involvement and depression. This does not mean that religious persons never get depressed or that nonreligious people are always depressed but only that persons who are more religious tend, on average, to be less depressed. In a review of research conducted prior to the year 2000, fifty-nine of ninety-three studies (63 percent) found lower rates of depressive disorder or fewer depressive symptoms among those with stronger religious beliefs or more frequent religious practices.[5] Of these ninety-three studies, most were cross-sectional studies (analyzing the relationship between religious involvement and depression at one point in time), but there were also twenty-two prospective cohort studies (examining whether religious involvement at an earlier time predicts less future depression) and eight randomized clinical trials (testing whether religious interventions reduce depression).

Among the twenty-two studies that followed subjects over time, fifteen found that greater religiousness predicted fewer depressive symptoms later on. Two of these studies diagnosed patients with a depressive disorder or significant depressive symptoms and followed them over time. Both of these studies found that depression resolved more quickly among more religious subjects. Of the eight clinical trials, five showed that depressed patients receiving religious-based interventions recovered faster than controls or those receiving a secular intervention. Of the thirty-four studies (out of ninety-three) that did not report less depression among the more religious, only four found that being religious was associated with significantly more depression.[6]

A recent meta-analysis of 147 studies by Smith and colleagues (including nearly 100,000 subjects) found an average negative correlation between religion and depression of –0.10, which increased to –0.15 in moderately or highly stressed samples.[7] While this is not a large correlation, it is of the same magnitude as that seen for gender. From a clinical standpoint, this finding has considerable significance since the prevalence rate of depressive disorder in women is known clinically to be much higher than in men. Furthermore, individual studies in stressed populations, particularly hospitalized medical patients, demonstrate that religion can have a substantial effect on the time it takes patients to get better from the depression. I now review some of the studies in medical populations conducted by my research group at Duke University.

In the first of these studies involving 850 older men with medical or neurological illness hospitalized at a Veterans Administration hospital, the degree to which religion was relied on to cope (religious coping) was inversely correlated to both self-rated and observer-rated depression, independent of nine other covariates.[8] The relationship was significantly stronger in those with more severe disability (and under more stress). During the prospective phase of the project, where 202 men were followed after discharge for an average of six months, religious coping was the only patient characteristic that predicted lower future depression scores.

In our second study, we used an investigative tool developed by the National Institutes of Mental Health: the Diagnostic Interview Schedule. Using this structured psychiatric interview, we identified eighty-seven hospitalized medical patients at Duke University

Medical Center with a depressive disorder.[9] Both men and women were included. These depressed patients were then followed for an average of forty-seven weeks, during which we examined baseline characteristics that might influence the speed of remission from depression after discharge (again, patients were on medical, not psychiatric wards). Religiousness was measured at baseline using the Hoge Intrinsic Religiosity Scale, which ranges in score from ten to fifty. We analyzed the data using Cox proportional hazards regression to examine the effects of intrinsic religiosity on depression outcome, independent of other characteristics. Results indicated that, for every ten-point increase on intrinsic religiosity, there was a 70 percent increase in the speed of remission. For patients who were not physically improving (i.e., had persistent or worsening physical disability), every ten-point increase on the Intrinsic Religiosity Scale predicted over a 100 percent increase in the speed of remission from depression. As in the first study of hospitalized male veterans, the effects of religious involvement appeared to be particularly strong in those who were experiencing greater psychological stress from severe physical disability. This finding is also consistent with the larger negative correlations between religion and depression in stressed populations reported by Smith and colleagues above (see note 7 in this chapter).

In the latest study by our group, we identified one thousand hospitalized medical patients with major and minor depressive disorder and followed 865 of these depressed patients for twelve to twenty-four weeks, examining factors that might influence the speed of remission from depression.[10] These patients were hospitalized with an acute worsening of either congestive heart failure or chronic lung disease, two conditions that have a very poor prognosis over time and are associated with marked disability and distressing physical symptoms. We identified the most religious subjects at baseline by a combination of religious beliefs and practices. Patients who attended religious services at least weekly, prayed at least daily, read the Bible or other religious scriptures at least three times weekly, *and* scored between forty-five and fifty on the Hoge Intrinsic Religiosity Scale (again, which ranges in total score from ten to fifty) made up 14 percent of the sample of 865 patients. After controlling for multiple demographic, psychosocial, psychiatric, and physical health predictors of remission, these patients (the most religious) got better from their depression over 50 percent faster than other patients.

Thus, studies in medical patients with serious and disabling medical conditions for whom little else can be done suggest that religious involvement is an important factor that may enable such patients to cope more successfully with stressful health problems. As indicated in the last chapter, religion is a powerful coping behavior whose effects are most easily demonstrated in populations experiencing stressors of some kind. Indeed, for nonstressed populations, one would not expect a coping behavior like religion to have much of an effect at all. This is not surprising since one would also not expect nondepressed people to report benefit from taking antidepressant medication. As with coping behaviors, medication is likely to make an observable difference only among those who have something to cope with.

Caregivers of family members with cancer are another high-risk group for depression, given the daily stress that they contend with twenty-four hours a day, living with and caring for a loved one with a condition that often leads to progressive disability, pain, and death. Fenix and colleagues at Yale University recently reported the results of a study that followed caregivers for thirteen months, examining associations between religiousness and the development of major depressive disorder in family caregivers of 175 patients with cancer who had recently died.[11] Religious caregivers were significantly less likely to develop major depressive order by the thirteen-month follow-up, a finding that persisted after adjusting for baseline depression, caregiver age, caregiver burden, and number of activities restricted due to the caregiving role. Religious caregivers were 26 percent less likely than others to develop major depression.

Critics say, however, that most of these studies are epidemiological. In other words, they are observational studies. In any observational study, it is always possible that there may be other characteristics that were not measured (and controlled for) that could explain the relationship between religion and depression. If that were indeed the case (i.e., called "confounding"), then it wouldn't be religion that was influencing the rate of depression but something else related to both religion and depression. Genetic factors have been hypothesized as one of these unmeasured factors. Perhaps religious people are simply genetically less likely to experience depression or more likely to be particularly hardy in recovering from depression.

In a fascinating study that examined the relationship of spirituality to serotonin ($5\text{-HT}_{1A}$) receptor binding in the brain using positive emission tomography, investigators found that $5\text{-HT}_{1A}$ receptor binding was *lower* in those who were more spiritually receptive (i.e., there was an inverse correlation between "spiritual acceptance" and $5\text{-HT}_{1A}$ receptor binding). A number of studies have shown that states of anxiety and depression are associated with *lower* $5\text{-HT}_{1A}$ receptor binding—the same pattern seen with spirituality.[12] Thus, if anything, spiritually oriented persons are biologically at *increased* risk for mood disorders, not at decreased risk. These findings argue against the notion that spiritually oriented persons are simply less prone to depression (if anything, the opposite appears to be true).

Besides epidemiological studies, however, there are at least eight randomized clinical trials of which five have shown a more-rapid remission of depression among patients receiving a religious-oriented psychotherapy.[13] Although these studies all involved religious subjects, at least they demonstrate that religious interventions in religious subjects (the vast majority of medical patients) result in faster improvement or remission of symptoms.

## SUICIDE

Suicidal thoughts, suicidal behavior, and completed suicide are indicators of poor mental health and often reflect an inability to cope with difficult circumstances, a loss of meaning and purpose in life, and feelings of overwhelming despondency and loss of hope. Suicide is most common at the age extremes, with the highest rates among the young and the old. For persons aged fifteen to thirty-four years, suicide is the third leading cause of death, and older adults have the highest suicide risk of all population groups. Because religious involvement helps persons to cope, provides meaning and purpose to life, and gives hope, and because most religions teach against suicide, one would expect there to be an inverse correlation between religiousness and suicide. Indeed, most published research indicates exactly this. Prior to 2000, there were sixty-eight studies of suicide rates or attitudes and level of religious involvement. Of those studies, fifty-seven found fewer suicides or more negative attitudes toward suicide among the more religious, nine showed no relationship, and two reported mixed results.[14] More recent research supports these findings and goes further to try to understand this relationship better.

For example, Van Tubergen and colleagues examined two possible explanations for the inverse correlation between religion and completed suicide: (1) religious networks provide support that reduces the emotional distress that can precipitate suicide, or (2) religious teachings prohibit suicide and so reduce its occurrence.[15] Investigators used individual and community-level data from the Netherlands on suicides committed between 1936 and 1973. Analyses were grouped into prewar and postwar periods in order to examine the effect of an increasingly secular Dutch society on this relationship. With an increasing proportion of religious persons in a city or region, they found that the likelihood of committing suicide decreased and that this was true for every denomination and for persons in those regions regardless of level of religious involvement. The effect among Protestants and Catholics was the same. The effect among believers and nonbelievers was the same. Comparing prewar and postwar periods, the protective effects of religion lessened as religious participation became less common in Dutch society. The authors concluded that religious participation has a general protective effect on suicide and that this comes primarily from religious prohibitions against suicide. As religious participation decreases in a society, they predicted that religious prohibitions have less and less of an effect.

Other research supports the important role that both religious prohibitions and religious support play in reducing suicide rates. For example, among 371 depressed psychiatric inpatients, religiously unaffiliated subjects had significantly more lifetime suicide attempts and more first-degree relatives who committed suicide than those who were religiously affiliated.[16] Furthermore, participants without a religious affiliation had both fewer reasons for living and fewer moral objections to suicide. Greening and Stoppelbein reported similar results from a study of over one thousand adolescents, who were asked to rate the likelihood that they would die by suicide.[17] Level of commitment to core religious beliefs (orthodoxy) emerged as the single strongest predictor after other risk factors were controlled for.

Besides prohibitions against suicide, the comfort and meaning derived from religious belief may also be relevant, particularly for those with medical illness. The protective effects of religion against suicide are most evident among those who are the sickest medically (similar to what is found for depression). For example, McClain and colleagues examined relationships between spiritual well-being, depression, and desire for death in 160 terminally ill cancer patients.[18] Investigators found that those with high spiritual well-being were significantly less likely to desire a hastened death, feel hopelessness, or have suicidal thoughts. In fact, when controlling for other predictors, spiritual well-being was the strongest predictor of each of the three outcomes, even stronger than depressive symptoms. Studies of this type, however, must be careful not to contaminate their measure of spiritual well-being with indicators of mental health.

## ANXIETY

Anxiety is an unpleasant, distressing feeling of fear or nervousness that can seriously interfere with quality of life and ability to function. Anxiety, like fear, often mobilizes people to make necessary changes in their lives in order to relieve this disturbing feeling. Unfortunately, it can also paralyze people so that they are unable to do anything. According to the U.S. Surgeon General's Mental Health Report in 1999, anxiety disorders are the most common mental health problem that Americans face, especially those over age fifty-five, where the prevalence is about one in ten (11 percent).[19]

There is an old saying that religion afflicts the comforted and comforts the afflicted. On the one hand, religious teachings cause guilt and fear that can help to motivate prosocial behavior that enhance relationships by encouraging forgiveness and altruistic activities and by discouraging behaviors that are harmful to others. On the other hand, religious beliefs and practices can comfort those who are fearful or anxious and return a sense of control (or reduce the need for personal control).

Prior to 2000, at least seventy-six studies examined the relationship between anxiety and religion, of which sixty-nine were observational and seven were randomized clinical trials.[20] Of the sixty-nine observational studies, thirty-five reported significantly less anxiety or less fear among the more religious, whereas twenty-four studies found no association and ten studies found greater anxiety. Greater anxiety? Indeed, religious teachings might evoke excessive fear and guilt in those who are already vulnerable because of underlying emotional illness. Consider, however, that the ten studies finding a positive relationship between religion and anxiety were all cross-sectional.

When examining studies like these that take a *cross-sectional* snapshot of this relationship at one point in time, it should not be surprising that those who are the most anxious are also those who are praying the most or otherwise involved in religious activities. Sayings such as "There are no atheists in foxholes" or "If you have nowhere to go, go to your knees" underscore this point. In that case, it is the anxiety that is causing the religious activity, not vice versa. While anxiety or fear may cause a person to turn to religion, religious activities may over time lead to a reduction in anxiety and a greater sense of peace (because it improves coping). When religious interventions are tested in religious persons with anxiety problems, these interventions actually lower anxiety. Of the seven clinical trials thus far completed, six found that the religious interventions reduced subjects' anxiety levels. More recent studies using Eastern spiritual techniques such as Buddhist "mindfulness" meditation likewise demonstrate such effects.[21]

Simply acknowledging that one is religious, however, may be less important than the extent to which religion is integrated into the person's life. Wink and Scott followed 155 subjects from middle age into later life (from their forties to late sixties or mid-seventies), examining the relationship between religiousness, fear of death, and dying in later life.[22] Although investigators found no linear relations between religiousness, fear of death, and dying, participants who were either high or low on religiosity had the lowest anxiety levels compared to those who were only moderately religious. Anxiety was particularly high among those who said that they believed in an afterlife but were not involved in religious practices. Investigators concluded that the firmness and consistency of religious involvement were more important in relieving death anxiety than was religiousness per se (or at least belief in an afterlife).

Certain forms of religious expression may be associated with greater, not lower, anxiety, particularly among those with serious medical illness. For example, a study of one hundred women with gynecological cancer examined the relationship between different kinds of religious coping and anxiety. Those women who felt that God was punishing them, had deserted them, or didn't have the power to make a difference, or who felt that their religious communities had deserted them (i.e., scored high on negative religious coping or religious struggles), had significantly higher anxiety levels than did other women, a result that persisted even after multiple statistical controls were taken into account.[23] These findings are consistent with other research showing greater emotional distress in medical patients with religious struggles or conflict.[24]

## WELL-BEING

In addition to research demonstrating an inverse relationship between religious involvement and emotional distress, there are also numerous studies reporting associations between religion and positive emotions. Most would agree that it is the positive emotions that make life truly worth living. Prior to 2000, my colleagues and I located one hundred studies that had examined links between religiousness and measures of well-being such as life satisfaction, happiness, positive affect, or high morale. Of those studies, close to 80 percent found that religious persons had significantly greater well-being than those who were less religious.[25]

Religion may lead to greater well-being through a number of pathways. It may do so by fostering hope, optimism, and joy, by increasing social support, and by giving life purpose and meaning. As with symptoms of emotional disorder described above, relationships between religion and positive emotions are especially likely to be detectable in persons undergoing stressful circumstances. Recent studies suggest that this is particularly true among stressed university students, older adults, those with medical illness, and persons from ethnic minority groups. For example, Salsman and colleagues reported that optimism and social support were key factors in explaining the greater adjustment due to religion in two samples of university students.[26] From the other end of the age spectrum, Krause analyzed data from a nationwide survey of older adults, finding that those who derived meaning in life from religious beliefs and practices had significantly higher levels of life satisfaction, self-esteem, and optimism, with effects strongest in African Americans.[27]

The connection with positive emotions can be particularly important for patients seen in medical settings, where religious involvement may influence well-being, life satisfaction, and satisfaction with medical care by enhancing ability to cope with physical illness. For example, Krupski and colleagues studied relationships between spirituality (measured using the Functional Assessment of Chronic Illness Therapy Spiritual Well-Being Scale [FACIT-sp]) and quality of life in a sample of 222 indigent men with prostate cancer.[28] Consistent positive associations were found between spirituality and quality of life; men with low spirituality had poorer adjustment and lower levels of well-being than those with high spirituality. Likewise, in a study of seventy-four hemodialysis patients with kidney failure, Berman and colleagues found intrinsic religiosity was strongly associated with life satisfaction in general, and greater involvement in religious community activities was associated with greater satisfaction with medical care.[29]

Again, because many of these studies are cross-sectional, it is not possible to determine whether religious participation increases psychological well-being or whether psychological well-being increases religious involvement. On the one hand, people who are unhappy may not wish to involve themselves in religious activities. On the other hand, religious involvement may increase well-being through the mechanisms described above, and studies that follow people over time tend to favor the latter explanation. Nevertheless, it is likely that both of these dynamics are true to some extent.

## Optimism and Hope

Optimism and hope are positive emotions that motivate and energize people facing difficult, stressful, burdensome situations. When everything is going well, life is naturally hopeful and optimistic.

When things are not going so well, positive emotions may decrease or disappear and are consciously sought after. In a review of the literature before the year 2000, twelve of fifteen studies that examined relationships between religious involvement and hope or optimism reported significant positive relationships, and effects were strongest in the studies with the best research designs.[30] Religious teachings often promote a positive view of the world that encompasses this life and the life thereafter. Religious scriptures provide the hope that good things can come out of every difficult situation and that all things are possible.

Recent studies on optimism suggest that such associations are particularly strong among those with serious or life-threatening illnesses and their caregivers. For example, the dispositional component of optimism (a general expectation of good outcomes) was greater in patients more likely to use prayer as a coping strategy prior to cardiac surgery.[31] Likewise, in a study of 450 patients with HIV/AIDS, religious/spiritual activities were associated with greater optimism concerning prognosis and life in general.[32] In contrast, negative religious coping or religious struggle was related to lower optimism in 162 caregivers of patients with terminal cancer.[33] The correlation between religion and optimism appears to be strongest in older adults and in African Americans.[34]

Recent studies also affirm the role that spirituality and religion play in maintaining hope, especially in the setting of physical illness or substance abuse. In two studies, McClain-Jacobson and colleagues found that spirituality predicted greater levels of hope among 160 cancer patients with only three months to live.[35] Likewise, Ironson and colleagues found significant correlations between religious/spiritual involvement and hope in two hundred HIV-positive patients in Miami.[36] Prayer as a coping strategy was also associated with greater hope in 226 patients prior to cardiac surgery, independent of other factors (especially the agency component of hope that involves the expectation that one can do something to make a difference). Studies of psychiatric patients have demonstrated similar relationships. In a study of twenty-one opioid-dependent substance abusers, a common theme involved the usefulness of spiritual interventions in reducing the hopelessness so common in this condition.[37] In a study of 115 patients in Switzerland with schizophrenia, 71 percent of patients reported that religion gave them hope, purpose, and meaning.[38]

## CONCLUSIONS

Much of the research on religion and mental health is cross-sectional and observational, making the argument for causality—that religion produces better mental health—less than airtight. For example, individuals with negative emotional states are perhaps less likely to seek religious involvement, which could explain some of the cross-sectional findings. Furthermore, there is little doubt that religion can also produce negative effects in vulnerable people, such as unhealthy guilt, increased fear, or worsening depression. Nevertheless, the evidence overall favors a positive impact for religion on mental health. Studies show consistent inverse correlations between religious involvement and negative emotions, such as depression and anxiety, while at the same time other studies report positive associations with positive emotions such as well-being, hope, and optimism.

These relationships are strongest among persons undergoing stress, especially the stress of medical illness, as would be expected if religion were an effective coping behavior. Prospective studies in medical patients show that religious involvement—independent of other factors—predicts faster remission of depression, and a number of randomized clinical trials now report that religious interventions speed the resolution of symptoms in those with depression or anxiety. These connections between religion and mental health may also have implications for physical health. The way we think, believe, and feel can affect our bodies. Now we move deeper into an examination of whether religion affects physical health as well.

# CHAPTER 6
## The Immune and Endocrine Systems

FOR MRS. HARRIS to live more than a century, her immune and endocrine systems must have been strong. They fought off infections, prevented or contained malignant processes, enabled her to heal after accidents or surgeries, and protected her from other diseases that commonly end life. Without these systems operating normally, none of us would live very long. The 1976 movie *The Boy in the Plastic Bubble*, starring John Travolta, dramatized how a boy without a fully functioning immune system ("severe combined immune deficiency") had to live in containers throughout his life. These "bubbles" shielded him from bacteria or viruses that would otherwise kill him. Unlike this boy, Mrs. Harris had particularly robust immune and endocrine systems—either because of genetic makeup, lifestyle, or attitude (or some of each) that kept these natural healing systems strong.

Mrs. Harris's resistance to disease might have also been aided by her religious faith, if what we have seen in the preceding chapters is true. Religion helps people cope, and it generally produces positive rather than negative emotions—which may affect positively immune and endocrine functions, as numerous studies show (see chapter 3). Now we look more closely at the relationships among religion/spirituality and these physical functions, especially among people who suffer weaknesses in this area: older adults and those with immune and endocrine disorders, such as people with the HIV infection or AIDS, autoimmune disorders, or metastatic cancer. The vulnerability of these persons to psychosocial stress shows up rapidly and clearly, compared to attempts at observing healthy subjects over many decades.

Psychosocial factors have an effect on two areas of immunity, (1) humoral and (2) cellular.[1] Humoral immunity consists of B lymphocytes secreting antibodies (also called immunoglobulins) in response to bacteria, viruses, abnormal cells, or other substances recognized as foreign. Cellular immunity involves cells that directly attack outside invaders or abnormal tissues (cancer) or help other cells to attack them. These include "natural killer" (NK) cells, antigen-specific cytotoxic T lymphocytes, and substances secreted by white blood cells called cytokines (inflammatory proteins). Humoral and cell-mediated immunity work together to protect the body, speed recovery from illness, and speed the healing of wounds or other damaged tissues.

The neuroendocrine system works in close coordination with the immune system, and there is an intricate feedback loop that enables each of these systems to influence and regulate one another. The primary hormone that affects immune functioning is cortisol, and this hormone is very sensitive to levels of psychological and social stress. Therefore, the simplest explanation for the stress response is that psychological stress (especially chronic stress) increases serum cortisol, which in turn, suppresses immune functions. As noted in chapter 3, however, things are a lot more complicated than that (since chronic stress may also exhaust cortisol secretion). For this chapter, however, I will keep things simple. A number of studies have examined the links among religious/spiritual practices, humoral and cellular immunity, and stress hormones, particularly cortisol. I review them below.

## HUMORAL IMMUNITY

The first study examining antibodies and religion was done by David McClelland in the department of psychology at Harvard University.[2] There are five major classes of immunoglobulins (antibodies) that are produced by B lymphocytes. These five are called: IgA, IgD, IgE, IgG, and IgM. The first, IgA, is an antibody found primarily in saliva. It protects the mouth and other mucous membranes in the gastrointestinal tract and lung from infection by bacteria or viruses—and IgA is where McClelland focused. He conducted an experiment to test whether the emotional arousal caused by watching a Mother Teresa film on caring for the poor had a different effect on salivary IgA compared to the emotions elicited by watching a movie of the human atrocities committed by Germany prior to World War II. His sample involved 132 college students who were experimentally assigned to the different films. The experiment was completed twice, once in the main sample and then repeated in a subsample. Results indicated that salivary IgA levels were significantly higher in those watching the Mother Teresa film (versus the World War II film) in both experimental trials. Although this study does not directly examine the relationship between religious involvement and humoral immunity, it does suggest that focusing attention on spiritual-type altruistic activities may have a positive impact on humoral immunity.

In another study, Harner examined the effects of shamanic drumming and "journeying" on salivary IgA levels in forty shamanic practitioners.[3] Shamanic drumming and journeying are spiritual practices originating in Siberia among traditional healers, and dating back over twenty thousand years to prehistoric times. They involve interacting with and traveling in the spirit world and are part of many native Indian practices in different areas of the world. For the Harner study, blood samples were drawn at baseline, during a resting state, during what the Siberian tradition calls a spiritual "birdsong" condition, and then after journeying/drumming. No differences in IgA levels were found between any of these conditions.

Most recently, Davidson and colleagues examined the effects of Buddhist "mindfulness" meditation on antibody response to influenza vaccine in twenty-five healthy employees of a biotechnology corporation in Madison, Wisconsin.[4] Those receiving the intervention were compared to sixteen employees randomly assigned to a wait-list control group. The "mindfulness-based stress reduction" intervention involved weekly meetings for two-and-a-half to three hours for eight weeks, one hour per day of meditation at home, and participation in a seven-hour silent retreat held toward the end of the intervention. At the end of the eight-week trial, both intervention and control groups were vaccinated with influenza vaccine, and blood was drawn at four and eight weeks afterward to examine antibody titers. Those in the "stress reduction" intervention group had a significantly greater rise in antibody titers from four to eight weeks after vaccination compared to the wait-list control group. Investigators concluded that this was the first study to report a reliable effect of meditation on an *in vivo* measure of immune function (antibody response).

## Cellular Immunity

Besides antibody production, the immune system also has cells that directly attack and engulf foreign pathogens or abnormal tissues. There is a fine balance, however, between cells that facilitate (T-helper cells) or suppress (T-suppressor cells) these immune reactions. Excessive facilitation could result in autoimmune disorders or life-threatening allergic reactions, whereas excessive suppression could result in an ineffective and underactive immune system. When we are healthy, these processes carefully balance out one another. Several studies suggest that religious involvement influences cellular immune processes and related immune proteins, such as cytokines.

### T-helper (CD4) Cells
The number of CD4 cells is a key measure of immune function in HIV-positive patients, since progression to AIDS is diagnosed when the CD4 count drops below two hundred per cubic

millimeter; furthermore, the likelihood of death increases substantially when CD4 counts drop below fifty. CD4 cells are also important in patients with malignancy, since they serve to help other cells destroy and contain cancer cells.

In the first study to examine religion-immune associations in HIV-positive patients, Woods and colleagues at the University of Miami examined the relationship between religious practices and immune function in 106 HIV-positive gay men.[5] Religious behaviors (measured by prayer, religious attendance, spiritual discussions, and reading religious/spiritual literature) and religious coping were assessed. Immune function was measured by CD4 cell counts and CD4 cell percentages. Religious behaviors were positively and significantly related to greater CD4 counts. Further analyses revealed that this relationship was not confounded by disease progression that may have prevented religious activities. Religious coping (putting trust in God, seeking God's help, and increased praying) was related to significantly fewer depressive symptoms as measured by the Beck Depression Inventory and tended to be related to less anxiety, but was unrelated to CD4 count (at least with religious behaviors in the statistical model).

Next, investigators at Stanford University examined relationships between religious involvement and immune function in women with metastatic breast cancer.[6] Spiritual expression was measured by the question, "How important is religious or spiritual expression in your life?" Attendance at religious services was assessed with the question, "How frequently do you attend religions services or meetings?" Immune parameters measured were total lymphocyte and white blood cell counts, percents and absolute numbers of T cells (CD3), T helper cells (CD4/CD3), cytotoxic T cells (CD8/CD3), and NK cells (CD56). Social network size was also assessed. Demographic characteristics, cancer status, and medical treatment variables were also controlled for. Results showed that spiritual expression was positively related to white blood cell count, total lymphocyte count, total T cells, and helper T cells. Social network size, disease, and medical treatment variables could not explain these relationships and had little effect on reducing the strength of the correlations. Similar positive trends were found for attendance at religious services, although they failed to reach statistical significance, except for antigen-specific cell-mediated immunity, which was inversely related to attendance. Religious expression was unrelated to delayed-type hypersensitivity in this study.

In one of the most interesting reports published to date, Ironson and colleagues at the University of Miami examined the effects of changes in spirituality/religiousness following the diagnosis of HIV and the consequences that this change had on CD4 cell levels and viral load over the next four years.[7] The sample consisted of one hundred patients who tested positive for HIV. Following diagnosis, 45 percent reported an increase in spirituality/religiousness, 42 percent remained the same, and 13 percent reported a decrease in spirituality/religiousness. Hierarchical linear modeling was used to examine the effects of change in spirituality/religiousness over time with the outcome being slopes of individual patient change in either CD4 cells or viral load (amount of virus in the system) during follow-up.

The HIV patients who reported an increase in spirituality/religiousness after diagnosis had significantly less decrease in their CD4 counts and significantly less increase in viral load during the four-year follow-up. Results were independent of church attendance and initial disease status, medication use at every time point, age, gender, race, education, health behaviors, depression, hopelessness, optimism coping, and social support. In fact, among all other predictors of CD4 cell preservation and viral load, change in spirituality/religiousness was the most powerful predictor. Religious service attendance was also an independent predictor in the same direction as increased spirituality/religiousness, but the effect was weaker.

## Natural-killer and Cytotoxic Cells

NK and cytotoxic T cells are lymphocytes that attack and destroy cancer cells and may help to limit cancer spread. As described earlier, a Stanford University study examined the relationship between religious involvement and immune function in women with metastatic breast cancer. These investigators found positive associations between religious expression and numbers of cytotoxic T cells. They reported a trend for greater NK-cell numbers as well.[8]

Another study of an Eastern religious practice—Qigong—also examined the association with NK cells. Qigong involves training in posture, breathing, movement, and focusing of attention. It relies on traditional Chinese religious beliefs concerning the "energy field" generated by the body or Qi (Ch'i), which is similar to Prana in Hindu yoga practice. Kimura and colleagues examined the effects on NK-cell activity of the Nishino Breathing Method, a breathing technique used to develop Qi (energy or life force), in twenty-one practitioners.[9] This method has a number of similarities with Qigong practice, including the use of visualization of the body Qi, slow body movements, and emission of Qi from one's hand. Blood levels were drawn before and after ninety minutes of practicing this method. Results indicated that NK-cell activity significantly increased between baseline and after the exercise and was increased in 76 percent of subjects. This finding corresponded with a reduction in level of stress as measured by the Lorish Face Scale method. Again, as in many other studies of this type, subjects were experienced practitioners of the method. Qigong and meditation have also been reported to increase T-cell count, although information on that study is limited.[10]

Yoga has also been studied. Kamei and colleagues examined changes in alpha brain rhythms and NK-cell activity before and after three yoga exercises (asana—postural changes, pranayama—breathing exercises and meditation) in eight experienced yoga instructors.[11] No relationships were found between alpha rhythms and NK activity for the asana or meditation periods, but there was a significant positive correlation between alpha rhythms and NK activity after fifteen minutes of *pranayama* breathing exercises. Investigators concluded that improved immune function may be achieved by activation of alpha rhythms during breathing exercises.

### Interleukin-6 (IL-6)

IL-6 is a blood protein called a cytokine that can influence cell-mediated immunity (see chapter 3). Persons with weakened immunity, such as those with AIDS, older adults, and those with certain cancers, have high levels of IL-6.

In the first study to examine the associations between religious activity and an indicator of immune function, researchers measured IL-6 and other biological indicators of inflammation in 1,718 participants in the Established Populations for Epidemiologic Studies in the Elderly (EPESE) study, funded by the National Institutes of Health.[12] Although religious attendance in 1986 and 1989 were unrelated to IL-6 levels in 1992, a significant inverse correlation was found between religious attendance in 1992 and IL-6 levels in 1992. Subjects who attended religious services were 49 percent less likely than nonattenders to have IL-6 levels greater than 5 pg/ml (a level above which is considered "high" for IL-6). When age, sex, race, education, chronic illness, and physical functioning were controlled, the effect was reduced from 49 percent to 42 percent but remained statistically significant.

Seven years later, Lutgendorf and colleagues in the department of psychology at the University of Iowa examined the effects of religious attendance on IL-6 levels in 556 older adults in the Iowa 65+ Rural Health Study, also part of the EPESE project.[13] Frequent church attendees (attending religious services more than once weekly) had IL-6 levels that were 66 percent lower than those of nonattendees. Frequent attendees also experienced a 68 percent reduction in mortality during the twelve-year follow-up, compared to nonattendees. When structural equation modeling was used to control for other predictors of mortality (including multiple measures of health status), lower IL-6 levels appeared to explain the relationship between religious attendance and mortality. This study suggests that IL-6 (reflecting immune function) mediated the relationship between religious attendance and lower mortality. This would be consistent with the hypothesized mechanism of religion's effect discussed in chapter 4—i.e., that religion is a coping behavior that reduces psychological and social stress and thereby enhances immune function, which then affects health status.

Most recently, Jacobson examined relationships between spirituality, religiosity, depression, and levels of IL-6 in a much smaller sample of seventy-three patients with terminal cancer.[14] Although no significant correlations were found between IL-6 and spirituality (using the Functional Assessment of Chronic Illness Therapy Spiritual Well-Being Scale), religiosity (using the Age Universal I/E Scale), or depression (using the Hamilton Depression Rating Scale) in the overall sample, correlations were moderate in size and in the expected directions for a small group of seven subjects who had their blood drawn within forty-eight hours of assessing spirituality, religiosity, and depression. Jacobson concluded that these findings were preliminary evidence that higher levels of spirituality and religiosity were associated with better immune function. Although this report by itself is hardly significant, if added to the other research findings above, it provides further evidence to support a connection between religion and IL-6.

By contrast, Yeager and colleagues examined data from a nationally representative survey of 944 older Taiwanese to assess the relationship between religious involvement and health status, including blood IL-6.[15] No relationship was found with religious beliefs or practices in this sample, composed mostly of participants affiliated with Taoist, traditional folk religion, or Buddhist traditions (in contrast to largely Christian samples in the earlier studies).

## Miscellaneous Immune Markers

Other studies have examined associations between a variety of religious or spiritual activities and immune measures. Neumann and Chi conducted a small study of thirty-eight healthy adults to explore the connection between church-related financial giving and immune function.[16] They compared those who gave 2 percent or less of their annual income ("Giving Little") with those who gave 9 percent or more ("Giving Much"). Giving was significantly correlated with religious attendance. Blood was drawn at three time points: baseline, after thirty minutes' rest, and after a standard five-minute stressor. The T-suppressor (CD-8) poststress levels increased more in the Giving Much group compared to the Giving Little group, a finding mirrored in the T-helper (CD-4)/T-suppressor (CD-8) cell ratios, which tended to decrease more in the Giving Much group after the stressor. This is significant in that patients with autoimmune disorders such as rheumatoid arthritis tend to have excessively high CD-4/CD-8 ratios, suggesting that those Giving Much may have some protection from autoimmune disorders. The Giving Little group also had significantly higher anger and hostility scores, lower forgiveness scores, and poorer stress-coping strategies than the Giving Much group.

Utilizing an Eastern religious intervention, Carlson and colleagues at the Baker Cancer Center in Calgary, Canada, examined the effects of "mindfulness" meditation (Buddhist prayer) on immune function and other outcomes in fifty-nine cancer patients (most with breast cancer).[17] Subjects received an eight-week "mindfulness-based stress reduction" program (MBSR) based on the work of Jon Kabat-Zinn. There was no control group. The intervention consisted of ninety-minute weekly group sessions along with home-based practice and a three-hour silent weekend retreat toward the end of the intervention. Subjects were excluded if they had previously participated in an MBSR group. (This is good, compared to many other studies of meditation that used experienced meditators.) Of the original fifty-nine subjects, seventeen dropped out for various reasons, so pre- and postmeasures were available on only forty-two subjects. Of thirty-three immune measures tested, seven significantly changed between pre- and postintervention. Monocytes, T-cell production of recombinant interferon gamma (both percentage of lymphocytes and total cell expression), and NK cell production of interleukin-10 (percentage of lymphocytes only) decreased from pre- to postintervention, while eosinophils and T-cell production of interleukin-4 (both percentage of lymphocytes and total cell expression) increased from pre- to postintervention. Psychological and immune change scores were unrelated. Overall, these findings did not fit a consistent pattern, and some may have been due to chance alone, given the multiple statistical comparisons.

## CORTISOL AND GROWTH HORMONE

In a review of the literature on religious/spiritual activities and neuroendocrine function prior to 2000, eleven studies were identified, most examining the effects of Eastern meditation.[18] Seven of nine studies found that Transcendental Meditation (TM), "mindfulness" meditation, or similar practices were associated with lower cortisol or better stress hormone levels. Two of eleven studies examined religious activities other than meditation. The first of these studied the relationship between religious coping and cortisol levels in thirty women awaiting breast biopsies for possible cancer. Those who employed prayer and faith to cope tended to have lower cortisol levels than those who did not, although this was only a descriptive study and no statistical comparisons were performed.[19] The second study (by Stanford researchers, described earlier) examined correlations between importance of religious or spiritual expression, frequency of religious attendance, and salivary cortisol levels in women with metastatic breast cancer.[20] Diurnal salivary cortisol levels were assessed over three consecutive days. Although overall salivary cortisol levels (area under the diurnal curves) were not associated with religious expression or attendance, evening cortisol levels were significantly lower among women reporting greater religious or spiritual expression.

Since 2000, several other studies have examined relationships between religious or spiritual practices and stress hormone levels. Ironson and colleagues examined the association between spirituality, religiousness, and long-term survival in patients with AIDS.[21] Spirituality/religiosity was measured using the Ironson-Woods Spirituality/Religiousness Index, which has four subscales (sense of peace, faith in God, religious behavior, and compassionate view of others). In this study, seventy-nine long-term survivors with AIDS were compared to a control group of two hundred HIV-positive patients. Results indicated that long-term survival was significantly related to all subscale scores and to frequency of prayer/meditation and religious attendance in the past month. Spirituality/religiosity was strongly and significantly related to less psychological distress, more hope, greater social support, better health behaviors, and altruistic behaviors. In particular, spirituality/religiosity was related to lower urinary cortisol levels. Further analyses revealed that the effect of spirituality/religiosity on long-term survival was mediated by low cortisol levels and by helping others with HIV (altruism).

Dedert and colleagues examined relationships between religiosity, spirituality, and diurnal salivary cortisol profiles in ninety-one women with fibromyalgia.[22] Religious involvement was measured using the Duke University Religion Index and Index of Core Spiritual Experiences. Results indicated that, controlling for age and medications, significant associations were found between diurnal cortisol rhythm, measures of private religious activity, and intrinsic religiosity. Moderately or highly religious patients had high morning and low evening salivary cortisol levels (reflecting a healthy rhythm). Patients with low religiosity had a flattened cortisol rhythm (not so healthy). Further analyses controlling for social support revealed that the relationship between cortisol rhythm (i.e., diurnal cortisol slope) and intrinsic religiosity remained significant, although the relationship with private religious activities weakened to a trend level.

Tartaro and colleagues from the Department of Psychology at Arizona State University investigated the associations between religiosity/spirituality and cortisol in a sample of young adults responding to a laboratory stressor under experimental conditions.[23] Again, they found that subjects scoring high on self-rated religiosity, self-rated spirituality, and frequency of prayer demonstrated lower cortisol responses to the stressor.

A number of recent studies have also examined the religion–stress hormone relationship in subjects from non-Christian religious traditions. Lee and colleagues at the Center for Integrative Medicine at Wonkwang University in Korea examined the effects of Qigong on immune function in a small sample of ten elderly male volunteers involved in Qigong training.[24] Blood was drawn before and after a one-hour session of Qigong. Differences in immune function (number of neutrophils) and endocrine function (growth hormone) before and after the session were compared. Growth-hormone levels increased significantly with the Qigong session. Oxygen production by neutrophils significantly increased from pre- to postsession (suggesting increased microbicidal activity). This effect was explained by the increase in growth hormone. However, it is not entirely clear why practicing Qigong would increase growth-hormone levels, since it is known that growth hormone increases in response to psychological stress[25] and Qigong has been shown to reduce stress levels by decreasing depression, hostility, and anxiety.[26]

Most recently (as described earlier), Yeager and colleagues examined data from 944 older Taiwanese on the relationship between religious involvement and health biomarkers, including urinary cortisol.[27] Unlike previous studies, over 92 percent of the sample was affiliated with non-Christian traditions, primarily Taoism/traditional folk religions and Buddhism. No relationship was found between religious beliefs or practices and cortisol level.

## CONCLUSIONS

Most studies demonstrating associations between religious or spiritual practices and immune or endocrine functions have been conducted in vulnerable populations, such as older adults, patients with advanced cancer, or those who are HIV-positive or have AIDS. The exception appears to be studies of Eastern meditation that are often done in healthy adults. Most studies are cross-sectional, although there are some impressive longitudinal studies (particularly those conducted at the University of Miami by Gail Ironson's group) and a number of clinical trials involving "mindfulness" meditation or Transcendental Meditation that report significant improvements in immune and endocrine functions. Many of the latter studies, however, were not randomized, and some involved experienced meditators without a control group.

Although much further research needs to be done, and research results are not always consistent, the evidence to date suggests that religious and spiritual behaviors are usually associated with better immune and endocrine functioning. This is true for Western religious practices and, to some extent, for Eastern religious practices as well.

## CHAPTER 7
## The Cardiovascular System

ONE OF THE BODY'S most sensitive areas to psychological and social stress is the cardiovascular system—the heart and blood vessels. The discussion of mechanisms and pathways in chapter 3 showed that the "fight-or-flight" response, caused by fear of some kind, produces physiological activity in this system in particular. These kinds of negative emotions (fear or anxiety) can arise from a sense of external threat or a sense of psychological threat.

Either way, the cardiovascular system responds by increasing heart rate and force of cardiac contractions, redistributing blood flow to muscles and brain, and pushing up blood pressure. As discussed in chapter 3, there is a close connection between stress and cardiovascular function. Furthermore, cardiovascular diseases are the most common cause of death in developed countries around the world, thus underscoring the need to understand relationships between religious involvement and cardiovascular functions.

The cardiovascular system is typically assessed by examining the heart (rate, rhythm, output, coronary blood flow) and the vascular system (blood pressure, thickness of blood-vessel walls). These may be measured at rest or after some kind of psychological or physical "stressor." Psychological stressors may involve tasks or activities that raise heart rate and blood pressure. Physical stressors may involve walking on a treadmill or engaging in some monitored physical activity. Most studies of religious/spiritual involvement and cardiovascular function involve large epidemiological studies—that is, surveys of the population—where religious/spiritual activities are assessed and a cardiovascular activity such as blood pressure is measured. In contrast, research done with "stressors" is less common. Studies using stressors have experimental designs. For example, this might involve measuring the religious/spiritual beliefs of subjects and then, after a stressful task over a short period, measuring blood pressure and heart rate. Using this approach, a number of clinical trials has examined the effects of spiritual interventions, most often Hindu or Buddhist forms of meditation, on cardiovascular functions.

In the next chapter (chapter 8), I will cover the large topic of cardiovascular *diseases*. My task now is more limited—to review four kinds of studies that relate religious/spiritual involvement to cardiovascular functions. These are (1) epidemiological studies of blood pressure, (2) experimental studies of cardiovascular reactivity, (3) clinical trials of interventions on lowering blood pressure, and (4) studies of how behaviors such as diet, exercise, and smoking influence cardiovascular functions.

## Epidemiological Studies

My colleagues and I at Duke University Medical Center have focused on epidemiology, the study of disease in large, relatively healthy populations. In our review of this literature published before 2000, we found sixteen studies that quantitatively examined the relationship between religion and blood pressure.[1] Of those studies, one found no association, one found a positive association (with self-rated religiosity), two found positive and negative associations, and the remaining twelve studies reported inverse associations. Of those twelve studies, eight studies reported statistically significant findings and four studies documented trends in that direction. Two of the studies were prospective, where subjects were followed over time.

In one of those studies, our team at Duke examined a random sample of 3,963 persons age sixty-five years or older participating in the NIH-funded Established Populations for Epidemiological Studies in the Elderly (EPESE).[2] After an in-home interview with our subjects, we measured their systolic and diastolic blood pressures following a standard protocol. Data from three waves of the EPESE survey (1986, 1989–90, and 1993–94) were used in analyses, which were also stratified by age (sixty-five to seventy-four versus over seventy-five) and by race (whites versus African Americans). Analyses were controlled for age, race, gender, education, physical functioning, body mass index, and, in prospective analyses, blood pressure from the previous wave. In cross-sectional analyses controlled for multiple covariates, those who both attended religious services at least once a week and prayed or studied the Bible at least once a day were 40 percent less likely to have diastolic blood pressures that equaled or exceeded 90 mm Hg (a number that indicates diastolic hypertension).

In the longitudinal part of the analyses, Wave II religious attendance predicted lower diastolic blood pressure in Wave III, after controlling for Wave II diastolic blood pressure and other factors that influenced blood pressure. When analyses were stratified by age and race, the findings were strongest in African Americans and younger elderly (ages sixty-five to seventy-four). In African Americans, Wave II religious attendance significantly predicted both diastolic and systolic blood pressures at Wave III, and Wave II private religious activity (prayer and Bible study) predicted lower diastolic blood pressures at Wave III. Although some of these findings may have been due to chance, given the multiple statistical tests, the pattern of results favored positive associations between religious variables and blood pressure in almost all analyses— except for watching religious TV, where some associations were reversed.

When the results of this study were reported in *Time* magazine, journalists emphasized the finding between watching religious television and *higher* blood pressure. Not long after that story was published, a minister contacted me requesting help for one of his parishioners. The minister said that, after reading the story in *Time*, a person in his congregation changed his last will and testament. Before that, the person had planned to leave his multimillion dollar estate to Trinity Broadcasting Corporation (a large religious television network). After reading the story, which emphasized religious television viewing and high blood pressure, he concluded that his high blood pressure was due to his watching religious programming and consequently changed his will. I had to clarify that this finding probably had other explanations than the one that *Time* magazine had emphasized. Older adults often have health problems (including problems with blood pressure) that prevent them from attending religious services. To compensate, they may turn to watching religious programs or listening to religious radio, which they can do in their homes. In such cases, it isn't the religious television that is causing the high blood pressure but the reverse—high blood pressure is causing health problems that prevent them from attending religious services, which they then compensate for by watching religion on television. The lesson here is not to take everything the media report at face value.

The second longitudinal study involved a twenty-year follow-up of 144 Catholic nuns who belonged to a secluded monastic order in Italy, comparing them to 138 laywomen controls living in a nearby town.[3] At the beginning of the study, average blood pressures in the two groups were equal. Over time, however, blood pressures increased gradually with age among the 138 laywomen controls but not among the Catholic sisters. The mean slope of the regression line for blood pressure was 0.89 in the nuns, compared to 2.17 in the laywomen, adjusting for other blood pressure risk factors. While investigators attributed this finding to the sisters' being isolated from the stresses of society, living closely with one another in a monastic order has its own unique stresses that the laywomen weren't exposed to. So I think that religious belief and commitment probably had a role in the slower increase of blood pressure with age among the nuns.

## Recent Studies

A number of new studies has been conducted since the review in 2000, many of which confirm the earlier findings. Research among minorities, where hypertension rates are high, has been particularly revealing.

For example, Yale University researchers examined associations between spiritual well-being, emotional distress, and blood pressure in a small sample of twenty-two African American women with Type II diabetes.[4] They reported significant inverse correlations between diastolic blood pressure and both total spiritual well-being and religious well-being.

Effects of race on the religion–blood pressure relationship were also the focus of a study of 679 African American women living on the east side of Detroit.[5] Multivariate analyses controlling for education, age, income, marital status, living situation, and physical functioning found that respondents who "prayed more" experienced fewer depressive symptoms but had more diabetes/hypertension. Those who "attended church more frequently" had better self-rated health, less diabetes/hypertension, and fewer depressive symptoms. Church-related social support mediated or explained some of these latter associations. Because of the cross-sectional nature of this study, it is difficult to determine the direction of causation in these somewhat conflicting findings (private religious activities associated with more hypertension, public religious activities associated with less).

In one of the few recent prospective studies, Steffen and Hinderliter studied the relationship between religious coping and blood pressure in 155 persons ages twenty-five to forty-five, half white Americans and half African Americans.[6] Primary outcome was twenty-four-hour ambulatory blood pressure and clinic-assessed blood pressure. Correlates measured included coping style, social support, depression, level of stress, and health behaviors. Regression analyses demonstrated an interaction between religious coping and ethnicity in their effects on blood pressure. In African Americans, but not whites, religious coping was inversely related to ambulatory blood pressure, independent of other correlates. Satisfaction with social support did not mediate this relationship. Thus, a consensus is building from previous and more recent studies that suggest an inverse relationship between religious involvement and blood pressure that is particularly strong among African Americans.

Such findings, however, are not restricted to minority groups. For example, Gillum and Ingram from the Centers for Disease Control and Prevention in Atlanta analyzed data from a random survey of 14,475 Americans, examining associations between frequency of religious attendance, history of hypertension treatment, and measured blood pressure.[7] Controlling for sociodemographic and health variables, those who attended religious services (regardless of ethnicity) had a lower prevalence of hypertension compared to nonattendees. Systolic blood pressure for weekly attendees was 1.5 mm Hg lower than nonattendees, and more than weekly attendees had systolic blood pressure of 3.0 mm Hg lower than nonattendees.

Although such blood pressure differences may seem minor and critics may question their clinical significance, research shows that cardiovascular risk increases with even small increases in blood pressure and that the majority of deaths from high blood pressure occur at pressures below treatment thresholds.[8] Furthermore, a reduction of a population's mean blood pressure by as little as 2–4 mm Hg could reduce cardiovascular disease by 10–20 percent.[9]

## Non-Christian Populations

Studies involving non-Christian populations have also been published since the year 2000. Krause and colleagues examined the ability of private religious practices, religious coping, and belief in an afterlife to reduce the negative effects of bereavement on hypertension in a Japanese population.[10] Researchers surveyed a random national sample of 1,723 older persons in Japan between 1996 and 1999. The survey included questions about religion, stressors (including bereavement), and health conditions (including hypertension). Results showed that belief in a good afterlife at the baseline interview buffered against the development of hypertension at follow-up.

By contrast, the study by Yeager and colleagues reviewed in the previous chapter that examined data from a nationally representative survey of older Taiwanese found that religious attendance was only weakly related to lower diastolic blood pressures and that there was no relationship between private religious activities and blood pressure, after controlling for multiple covariates.[11] As in the Japanese study above, this sample was composed primarily of non-Christian participants.

In the only study of the religion–blood pressure relationship from the Middle East, Al-Kandari examined blood pressure in a convenience sample of 223 Kuwaitis (mean age thirty years).[12] Sampling was done to ensure that there was adequate representation of both Sunni and Shiite Muslims and urban and Bedouin participants. Two nurses measured blood pressures on each individual until differences were less than 10 mm Hg on three separate occasions after averaging the readings for the three measurements. Religiosity was measured by a self-report of daily prayer and a fifteen-item scale assessing devoutness to Islam; these were combined to form a single religious commitment scale. Religious commitment was inversely related to systolic and diastolic blood pressures after controlling for age, gender, socioeconomic status, smoking, and body mass index.

In summary, epidemiological studies have included both cross-sectional and longitudinal research, random and nonrandom samples, subjects from Christian and non-Christian populations, and those from different ethnic backgrounds. These studies often, but not always, demonstrate associations between religious or spiritual activities and lower blood pressure.

## EXPERIMENTAL STUDIES

Studies of cardiovascular "reactivity" have enabled researchers to examine experimentally whether subjects' religious characteristics affect their cardiovascular responses. The reactivity of blood pressure to psychological stress has been studied in this regard. Blood pressure reactivity is known to be a strong predictor of later cardiovascular disease and has the potential to affect long-term health outcomes.[13]

In one of the first of these studies, investigators at Rutgers University reported that higher religiosity in a sample of younger adults was related to lower diastolic blood-pressure reactivity to a stressful speech task, but not to a mental arithmetic stressor.[14] Tartaro and colleagues from the University of Arizona also investigated associations between religion/spirituality and blood-pressure reactivity in a sample of young adults responding to a standard laboratory stressor.[15] They reported that greater total scores on self-rated religiosity and spirituality and frequency of prayer and attendance at services were all associated with lower blood pressure in males but with higher blood pressure in females. Investigators concluded that religion/spirituality may help to protect against the cardiovascular responses to stress, although the effects could vary by gender.

Finally, Masters and colleagues from Utah State University examined the relationship between religiosity (intrinsic versus extrinsic religiousness) and blood-pressure reactivity in a sample of 178 participants (75 older and 103 younger adults).[16] Subjects were divided up based on whether they had an intrinsic or extrinsic religious orientation, using the Religious Orientation Scale and were then exposed to cognitive and interpersonal stressors in the laboratory. Systolic and diastolic blood pressures were assessed at baseline and during the psychological stressors. Researchers reported that older subjects (ages 60 to 103) who were extrinsically religious had exaggerated blood-pressure reactivity during stressors, compared to both younger subjects (ages eighteen to twenty-four) and older intrinsically religious subjects. There was no difference in systolic blood-pressure reactivity between older intrinsically religious subjects and younger subjects. Again, effects were particularly notable for an interpersonal stressor that involved role-playing, compared to a mental arithmetic stressor. Those with intrinsic religious orientation had less systolic blood-pressure reactivity regardless of age. Effects were similar for diastolic blood pressure but not as pronounced.

## CLINICAL TRIALS

Randomized clinical trials are important because they have the ability to determine causality—in other words, they can answer the question "Do spiritual interventions cause a reduction in blood pressure?" In our earlier review of religion–blood-pressure studies, we identified nine clinical trials conducted before the year 2000 that tested the effects of a spiritual intervention on lowering blood pressure (Eastern meditation in all cases).[17] In seven of those nine studies, meditation significantly reduced blood pressures in the treated group. While most of these clinical trials were not randomized, two of the studies finding positive effects were randomized controlled studies.

In the first study, researchers at Maharishi University in Fairfield, Iowa, randomly assigned 111 African Americans in Oakland, California, ages fifty-five to eighty-five, with mild hypertension to Transcendental Meditation (TM), Progressive Muscle Relaxation, or a Stress Education Control group.[18] TM and Progressive Muscle Relaxation sessions lasted one-and-a-half hours initially and one-and-a-half hours per month for three months (and subjects practiced daily at home). Researchers reported that subjects in the TM group had significantly greater reductions of systolic blood pressure and diastolic blood pressure compared to those in the Progressive Muscle Relaxation group. Among subjects in the TM group, systolic blood pressure was reduced by 10.7 mm Hg, and diastolic blood pressure was reduced by 6.4 mm Hg, compared to the Stress Education Control group. In comparison, Progressive Muscle Relaxation reduced systolic pressure by 4.7 mm Hg and diastolic by 3.3 mm Hg (which was significantly smaller than the TM group). Overall, then, TM was twice as effective as Progressive Muscle Relaxation in reducing systolic and diastolic blood pressures.

In the second study, the same research group at Maharishi University examined the effects of TM on ambulatory blood pressure in thirty-nine men with normal blood pressure.[19] Subjects were randomized to either TM or a Stress Education Control control group. After four months of TM, intervention and control subjects were compared. Although there was no change in cardiovascular response to stressors between intervention and control groups, subjects in the TM group who were compliant in practicing TM experienced a significant 9 mm Hg reduction in mean ambulatory diastolic blood pressure, compared to those in the control group. Although this was a negative study overall, it suggests that those who actually meditate on a regular basis may receive benefit in terms of blood-pressure reductions.

### Recent Studies

In the third and most recent study by the Maharishi University researchers, investigators used the same design as the first study above but extended the intervention to twelve months and increased the sample size to 150 African American men and women with an average age of forty-nine and an average blood pressure of 142/95.[20] Recruited from a community health center, subjects were randomized to TM, Progressive Muscle Relaxation, or a Stress Education Control group. The intervention consisted of an introductory and preparatory lecture, a brief interview, a sixty- to ninety-minute session of personal instruction, and three ninety-minute follow-up sessions taking place during three consecutive days. Subjects were instructed then to practice at home for twenty minutes twice a day. After twelve months, members of the TM group decreased their systolic blood pressure by 3.1 mm Hg and their diastolic blood pressure by 5.7 mm Hg, compared to members of the Progressive Muscle Relaxation group, who reduced them by 0.5 and 2.9 mm Hg, respectively. The difference between TM and Progressive Muscle Relaxation groups was not significant for systolic blood pressure but was for diastolic blood pressure. Furthermore, the TM group was able to reduce use of antihypertensive medication compared to the Progressive Muscle Relaxation group, and there was a similar trend compared to the Stress Education Control group. Effects were greater in women than in men. Subjects enrolled for this study were not experienced meditators.

Other research groups besides the one at Maharishi University have conducted clinical trials on the effectiveness of spiritual practices on cardiovascular functions. For example, Harinath and colleagues examined the effects of Hindu Hatha yoga and Omkar meditation on cardiovascular measures in thirty healthy young adult male volunteers (without experience in yoga or meditation).[21] Subjects were randomized to either the intervention (yogic postures, breathing exercises, and meditation) or a control group (flexibility exercises, slow running, playing video games), which they performed for two hours each day. Subjects in the intervention group dropped their systolic, diastolic, and mean arterial blood pressures over the three months of the study by nearly 10 mm Hg, while members of the control group experienced little fluctuation in blood pressure.

Finally, Paul-Labrador and colleagues (in collaboration with investigators from Maharishi University in Fairfield, Iowa) examined the effects of TM on cardiovascular and metabolic functions in a sample of patients with coronary artery disease (CAD).[22] They randomized 103 patients with stable coronary artery disease to either TM or a Stress Education Control group for sixteen weeks. Subjects were excluded if they had performed TM or stress management in the past. The TM protocol consisted of two ninety-minute introductory lectures, a brief personal interview, one ninety-min-ute personal instruction, three ninety-minute group meetings, two ninety-minute maintenance group meetings per week for the first four weeks, and one ninety-minute maintenance meeting per week thereafter (along with twice-daily TM sessions practiced at home). Control subjects had discussions of the effects of stress, diet, and ex-ercise on CAD during their group meetings and were given home-work assignments lasting the same amount of time as the home TM sessions. Results indicated that those in the TM group expe-rienced a significant 3.4 mm Hg reduction in systolic blood pres-sure compared to a 2.8 mm Hg increase in controls. The TM group also tended to have greater heart-rate variability (which is good). There was no difference between groups in diastolic blood pres-sure or in brachial-artery reactivity testing (which measures blood flow in the brachial artery after withdrawal of blood-pressure-low-ering medications).

There is even research suggesting that spiritual interventions may reverse the atherosclerotic changes responsible for arterial-wall thickness, which is a known risk factor for coronary artery dis-ease and stroke. For example, Castillo-Richmond and colleagues (again from Maharishi University) examined the effects of Tran-scendental Meditation (TM) on carotid artery intima-media thick-ness in a sample of sixty African Americans with hypertension.[23] Subjects were randomly assigned to either TM or a cardiovascular risk factor–reduction health-education control group. The clinical trial was conducted over six to nine months. Age and pretest intima-media thickness were controlled for in the analyses. The TM group experienced a significant decrease of 0.098 mm in intima-media thickness compared to an increase of 0.054 mm among controls.

There is also evidence that the rhythms of speaking and breath-ing that occur during spiritual practices may influence cardiovas-cular rhythms in a positive direction. For example, Bernardi and colleagues in Florence and Pavia, Italy, examined the effects of saying the rosary in Latin and repeating a yoga mantra in Hindu on autonomic and cardiovascular rhythms.[24] In other words, the rosary and the yoga mantra were recited in their original languages. Subjects were twenty-three healthy adults. Researchers reported that both recitation of the rosary and the mantras caused significant increases in cardiovascular rhythms when these prayers were recited six times per minute. There was a significant increase from 9.5 to 11.5 ms/mm Hg in baroreflex sensitivity, which has been associated with positive cardiac outcomes such as greater heart-rate variability.[25]

Some religious practices, however, are thought to increase blood pressure and possibly even cause hypertension. There is concern that the repetitive fasting (from sunrise to sunset) and eating (from sunset to sunrise) that Muslims engage in during the month of Ramadan may adversely affect blood pressure, especially in those with hypertension.[26] This is particularly true since repeated cycles of fasting and refeeding in animals have been shown to increase blood pressure to hypertensive levels. Muslim rituals during Ramadan may also involve altered sleep patterns and changes in the timing of taking medication. Perk and colleagues examined the effects of Ramadan fasting on ambulatory blood pressure in seventeen subjects taking antihypertensive medication.[27] Results of this study showed that mean blood pressure did not change during Ramadan, allaying concerns about the negative effect of such religious practices on blood pressure.

## HEALTH BEHAVIORS

Religious or spiritual activities are also associated with a host of health behaviors that influence cardiovascular function, such as diet (and cholesterol), exercise, and smoking.

### Diet

Special dietary practices play a major role in many if not all world religions, such as periods of fasting, sanctioning of certain foods, and prohibition against other foods. For example, Catholic and Orthodox traditions discourage eating meat on Fridays, and conservative Christian traditions may encourage fasting for religious reasons. Seventh-day Adventists are frequently vegetarian, and their average life expectancy exceeds that of the general population by an average of four years, with lower death rates from cardiovascular diseases, in particular.[28] Orthodox and some Conservative Jews adhere to a kosher diet, which excludes shellfish and pork, a practice that could affect blood lipid levels. As noted above, most Muslims practice daytime fasting during the month of Ramadan. Hindus and Buddhists likewise have their own rules related to diet.

These various dietary practices are known to affect a host of metabolic factors that influence cardiovascular functions. For example, investigators studied the effects of fasting during Ramadan on lipid and lipoprotein metabolism in thirty-two healthy adult male volunteers from Morocco.[29] Compared to the prefasting period, there was a 7.9 percent decrease in total serum cholesterol and a 30 percent decrease in triglycerides during Ramadan. By the end of Ramadan, HDL (good cholesterol) had increased by 14.3 percent and remained elevated for one month after the end of Ramadan. By contrast, LDL (bad cholesterol) decreased by 11.7 percent and remained low for one month after Ramadan. Furthermore, intake of dietary saturated fat decreased significantly during Ramadan, and mono- and polyunsaturated fat in the diet increased. All these changes suggest an improvement in lipid and lipoprotein metabolism as a result of dietary practices during Ramadan.

In an earlier study of nearly seven hundred seventeen-year-olds in Jerusalem, Friedlander and colleagues found that those from observant Jewish families had significantly lower serum cholesterol, triglyceride, and LDL levels compared to youth from secular families, controlling for gender, country of origin, social class, body mass index, and season.[30] Observant families were those who followed the religious commandments, kept kosher, abstained from travel on the Sabbath, attended synagogue, observed Jewish rituals, and reported a higher degree of orthodoxy. Investigators concluded that these findings could help to explain the lower rates of coronary artery disease found among religiously active Jews.

## Exercise

My colleagues and I identified five studies in our earlier review that quantitatively examined the relationship between religious involvement and exercise.[31] Three of those five studies found a positive relationship between religious involvement and exercise, one found no association, and one documented a negative relationship. Of these five studies, the best designed was a twenty-eight-year prospective study conducted by Strawbridge and colleagues at the Human Population Laboratory in Berkeley, California, that examined data collected during the Alameda County Study.[32] Investigators followed a random sample of 5,286 adults from 1965 to 1994, analyzing the relationship between religious attendance and health outcomes, including exercise. Frequent church attendees (once a week or more) were significantly more likely (38 percent) to increase exercise levels during follow-up, after controlling for age, gender, ethnicity, education, religious affiliation, chronic conditions, mobility impairment, perceived health, and depression. By contrast, the one study that found a negative correlation between religion and exercise was conducted in a sample of sixty-nine undergraduates and seven adult members of a Protestant church.[33] Intrinsic religiosity was inversely related to exercise. This was a simple cross-sectional correlation, and one of nearly 150 correlations performed without any other predictors of exercise controlled for. Due to the multiple comparisons, that finding could have easily been a statistical fluke.

In more recent studies, Kim and Sobal examined 546 adults in an upper New York state county, finding that religious characteristics were associated with greater physical activity in both women and men, although this depended on the particular religious characteristic.[34] Among women, greater religious commitment was associated with more moderate and vigorous physical activity, whereas, among men, "divine" social support was associated with greater physical activity.

In a study of 6,188 adults in Utah, investigators reported that those attending religious services weekly or more were significantly more likely to exercise at least twenty minutes three times per week compared to less frequent attendees.[35] This was explained in part by the lower likelihood of cigarette smoking and the better overall health of frequent church attendees. Church-based exercise programs, especially in minority populations, have been developed to increase exercise in order to reduce cardiovascular morbidity.[36]

### Smoking

Reviewing the research prior to 2000, we found twenty-five studies that had examined the religion-smoking relationship.[37] Of those, twenty-two found significant inverse correlations between religious involvement and cigarette smoking, two others reported trends in that direction, and one found no association. For example, my colleagues and I at Duke University Medical Center examined cigarette smoking in a random sample of nearly four thousand persons aged sixty-five or over.[38] Those who both attended religious services at least weekly and prayed or studied the Bible at least daily were almost 90 percent more likely not to smoke, compared to persons less involved in both these religious activities. Total number of pack–years smoked was also inversely related to frequency of religious attendance and to private religious activities. Retrospective and prospective analyses revealed that more religiously active persons were less likely ever to start smoking.

## Conclusions

There is evidence from cross-sectional studies, and to a lesser extent from prospective studies, that religious involvement or spiritual practices are related to lower blood pressure and less hypertension. These findings are reinforced by a few experimental studies that show lower cardiovascular reactivity in more religious subjects, although this effect may vary by gender. Clinical trials, including a number of randomized trials in relatively large samples, show that spiritual practices like meditation can lower blood pressure, reduce the need for antihypertensive medication, and may even reduce arterial wall thickness, a risk factor for coronary artery disease and stroke. Finally, other factors known to influence cardiovascular functions, such as exercise, diet, cholesterol, and cigarette smoking, all appear to be at healthier levels in those who are more religious or spiritually active.

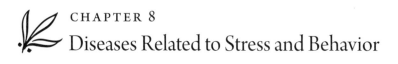

## CHAPTER 8
# Diseases Related to Stress and Behavior

FROM STUDIES reviewed earlier in this book, it appears that psychological stress and health-related behaviors are closely linked to a variety of physical diseases. I have argued that religious involvement may affect both psychological stress levels and health behaviors and, therefore, might naturally be expected to have some connection with diseases influenced by these factors. The focus of this chapter is on the relationship between religious involvement and *medical conditions* that are affected by psychological stress or health habits, such as coronary artery disease (myocardial infarction), cardiac surgery outcomes, stroke, dementia, diabetes, and cancer. Because space is limited, readers are referred to the *Handbook of Religion and Health* for a more extensive discussion.

## CORONARY ARTERY DISEASE

A number of studies have already been reviewed suggesting a relationship between religious involvement and cardiovascular functions. Surprisingly, however, few investigators have examined the association between religion and coronary artery disease (CAD), despite its obvious potential impact on public health. CAD is one of our most common medical problems and causes of death. Most of the research on CAD involves the role of religion in coping with heart disease, improving quality of life, and lowering the risk of depression. What we lack are studies of the effects of religious involvement on rates of CAD or disease outcomes. Besides the

Comstock studies in the early 1970s, very little research has been done on U.S. populations.[1] The most recent studies are from Israel and India, and at least one other examines the effects of Eastern meditation. In this discussion, I will not include any of the double-blinded intercessory prayer studies in cardiac patients, since I believe they have little scientific or theological credibility.[2]

In a case-control study, Friedlander and colleagues examined 454 men and 85 women following their first myocardial infarction, comparing them to a control group of 295 men and 391 women without CAD.[3] All subjects were under age sixty-five years, Jewish, and residents of Jerusalem. Based on responses to six questions and a question about self-rated religious orthodoxy, subjects were classified as orthodox, traditional, or secular. Results indicated that 51 percent of men and 50 percent of women in the postmyocardial infarction group defined themselves as "secular" compared with 21 percent of men and 16 percent of women in the control group. After adjusting analyses for age, ethnicity, education, smoking, physical exercise, and body mass index, investigators found that secular subjects still had a significantly higher risk of myocardial infarction compared to orthodox subjects. Secular males were over four times more likely to have had a myocardial infarction, whereas secular women subjects were over seven times more likely. This relationship persisted in a smaller sample of cases examined two to three months after the acute phase of the myocardial infarction, controlling for total cholesterol, HDL cholesterol, and blood pressure.

Next, Goldbourt and colleagues reported results from a prospective study of 10,059 Jewish males aged forty or over working as civil servants or municipal employees in Israel who were followed from 1963 to 1986 (twenty-three years).[4] Three questions were used to measure religious orthodoxy (religious versus secular education; self-definition as orthodox, traditional, or secular; and frequency of synagogue attendance); these were summed to create an orthodoxy index with five ranked categories. Religious data were available on 9,245 subjects. Those scoring high on the above orthodoxy index, who comprised 23 percent of the sample, had a significantly lower rate of mortality from both CAD (38 versus 61 per 10,000) and other causes (135 versus 168 per 10,000) compared to those who scored low on the orthodoxy index (19 percent of the sample). The risk of death from CAD during the twenty-three-year follow-up was at least 20 percent lower among the most orthodox group compared to other participants in the sample, and this effect was independent of age, blood pressure, cholesterol, smoking, diabetes, body mass index, and baseline CAD.

In a study that examined a rural Hindu population in India, Gupta and colleagues examined risk factors for CAD in 3,148 adults using a cross-sectional design.[5] Religious involvement was measured by participation in religious prayer or yoga, which 30 percent of the sample was involved in. Multivariate analysis showed that prayer was a significant, independent protective factor against CAD, reducing the risk of disease by over 70 percent.

In another study from India, Gopinath and colleagues surveyed a random sample of 13,560 adults of different ethnic groups in Delhi, examining prevalence of CAD (based on treatment history or electrocardiograph evidence) in various religious groups.[6] The prevalence rate of CAD per thousand adults was the highest in Sikhs (47.3 percent), lowest in Muslims (22.8), and identical in Hindus (31.8) and Christians (31.2). The prevalence rate of silent CAD based on electrocardiograph was highest in Muslims (89.5) and Sikhs (87.3), lowest in Christians (25.0), and intermediate in Hindus (60.0). Sikhs showed the highest prevalence of myocardial infarction (15.5) and of myocardial ischemia (31.8) compared to other religious groups. Researchers indicated that differences in prevalence rates by religious group could not be explained by conventional risk factors. In other research, Seventh-day Adventists have been shown to have lower rates of CAD than non-Adventists.[7] Dietary factors partially explain the different rates of CAD by religious group in these studies.

There are only a few clinical trials of religious or spiritual interventions in CAD. In one such study, investigators examined the effects of Transcendental Meditation (TM) on exercise-induced myocardial ischemia. Zamarra and colleagues from Maharishi University and SUNY at Buffalo recruited and assigned twenty-one patients with known CAD to either TM or a waitlist control group.[8] Five subjects did not complete the study, leaving only ten subjects in the test group and six in the control (all men, average age fifty-five years). The TM intervention consisted of ten hours of basic instruction, personal instruction for sixty minutes, and then thirty minutes twice per week for the first month and monthly thereafter. In addition, subjects practiced TM twice daily for twenty minutes each time. After eight months, TM patients had a 14.7 percent increase in exercise duration, an 11.7 percent increase in maximal workload, and an 18.1 percent delay of onset in ST segment depression (a measure of low blood circulation in the coronary arteries), whereas control subjects showed no substantial changes in these outcomes. Note, however, that these analyses were before-and-after comparisons (not comparison of TM versus controls), and there was no evidence for random assignment (both serious study flaws).

There are also some dissenting studies. Measuring religious coping in terms of self-directing ("God grants me freedom to solve my own problems myself"), collaborative ("God and I actively work together to solve my problems"), and deferring ("I turn my problems over to God and wait for his solutions to emerge), Yelsma and Montambo found no relationship between religious coping style and recovery from acute myocardial infarction in a small sample of fifty-five medical patients and spouses one to forty-eight months after completing a rehabilitation program in Michigan.[9] In a prospective study of seventy male Hindu patients interviewed four to five days after their first heart attack, Agrawal and Dalal inquired about patients' world beliefs, causal beliefs, and recovery beliefs concerning their conditions, and then subjects were reassessed one month later.[10] Three domains of beliefs were examined: karma,

God, and just world (or self). Outcomes assessed were physical and psychological recovery. Investigators reported that attributing causality to God was *negatively* correlated with medical recovery, perceived recovery, and mood state on follow-up.

Thus, there is evidence from large epidemiological studies in persons from a variety of religious groups that religious involvement is associated with a lower risk of myocardial infarction and CAD. There is also some evidence from a nonrandomized clinical trial that Hindu meditation reduces exercise-induced myocardial ischemia. On the other hand, not all studies find positive associations between religious or spiritual beliefs and a lower risk of or faster recovery from myocardial infarction, and much further research is needed.

## Cardiac Surgery Outcomes

If religious or spiritual factors influence coping with illness, reduce stress levels, positively impact immune and endocrine processes, and improve cardiovascular responses, then recovery rates from surgery ought to be likewise affected. This is particularly true since wound closure and infection rates depend heavily on immune, endocrine, and cardiovascular functions. At least three studies have examined the relationship between religious involvement and outcomes following open-heart surgery.

Oxman and colleagues at Dartmouth prospectively followed 232 patients for an average of six months following elective cardiac surgery for coronary artery bypass grafting, heart-valve replacement, or both, examining relationships between religious involvement and mortality.[11] Religious characteristics assessed at baseline included religious affiliation, attendance at services, strength and comfort from religion, number of people known in congregation, and self-rated religiousness. Statistical analyses controlled for previous cardiac surgery, severity of impairment in baseline physical functioning, age, and participation in social groups. Subjects who indicated a lack of strength or comfort from religion had a mortality risk that was three times greater than other patients. Among seventy-two patients who had both high social group participation and high religious strength and comfort, only 2.5 percent died, compared with over 21 percent of the forty-nine subjects with no group participation or deriving no comfort from religion.

In a second study, Contrada and colleagues from Rutgers University prospectively followed 142 patients before and after heart surgery, examining factors affecting hospital stay and complication rates.[12] Religiousness (measured by a five-item scale assessing degree of religiousness, a single item assessing religious attendance, and a single item assessing private prayer) and other psychosocial factors (depressive symptoms, social support, optimism, anger/hostility) were assessed one week prior to surgery. Outcomes were length of hospital stay and complications, which were determined based on hospital chart review following surgery. Greater religiousness predicted fewer postsurgical complications and shorter hospital stays. Frequency of prayer did not predict either complications or length of hospital stay. Frequency of attendance at religious services was unrelated to complications but paradoxically predicted *longer* hospital stays (the opposite of religiousness). Effects of religiousness were stronger in women than men and were independent of biomedical and other psychosocial predictors.

Finally, Ai and colleagues prospectively examined the effects of depression and religious coping on postoperative global functioning following cardiac surgery in 335 patients assessed both before and after surgery.[13] Regression analyses revealed that preoperative positive religious coping predicted better postoperative functioning, even after controlling for preoperative depression and other patient characteristics. Postoperative prayer frequency, however, was associated with worse postoperative functioning, although this may have been due to patients' turning to prayer as a result of poor function or a complicated postoperative course.

These studies, then, suggest that religious beliefs and practices can influence the course of illness following cardiac surgery, including overall survival, postoperative complications, length of hospital stay, and ability to function, at least in certain populations.

## STROKE

If research suggests that blood pressure is related to religious involvement, then, since hypertension is the most common cause of stroke, it would be reasonable to expect lower rates of stroke among those who are more religious. This is particularly true since research reviewed previously suggests that spiritual practices such as Transcendental Meditation may actually reduce carotid artery wall thickness, which is a major cause of stroke.[14]

Research shows that rates of stroke differ by religious group. Mormons and Seventh-day Adventists are known to experience lower stroke rates than persons with other religious affiliations or no affiliation.[15] Although these findings have been explained in terms of diet and lifestyle, they are a consequence of particular religious beliefs and practices.

In one of the few studies that has prospectively examined the effects of religious activity on stroke risk, Colantonio and colleagues at Yale University followed 2,812 persons over age sixty-five for a seven-year period.[16] During that time, 167 new strokes occurred. In the uncontrolled analysis, higher depression scores (using the Center for Epidemiologic Studies-Depression scale) and less religious attendance predicted a greater stroke risk. Religious coping and self-rated religiosity were unrelated to stroke incidence. When age, gender, hypertension, diabetes, physical function, and smoking were controlled for, the significant associations between stroke rate and both attendance and depression disappeared.

These analyses, however, did not distinguish between confounders and explanatory variables. Since the effect of religious involvement on stroke is most likely caused by effects on blood pressure and health behaviors, we can expect that, when hypertension and behaviors such as smoking are controlled, the effects will disappear. These mediating factors explain how religion may affect stroke rate and controlling for them does not invalidate the results. Besides this single study, no other research has examined whether religious involvement is related to stroke risk. There is evidence, however, that chronic illnesses like stroke can influence religious activity, such as religious attendance, so the relationship may be bidirectional.[17]

## DEMENTIA

Several studies suggest that religious involvement may forestall the development of cognitive impairment in older adults and may even influence the progression of Alzheimer's disease. Although the mechanism remains unclear, it is likely related to the effects that psychological stress and depression have on cognitive functioning through endocrine pathways (see chapter 3).

In the first study to report such an association, Van Ness and Kasl at Yale University examined cognitive dysfunction and religious involvement in a random sample of 1,847 community-dwelling older adults (over age sixty-five) in New Haven, Connecticut.[18] They measured religious attendance in 1982 to see if it could predict cognitive dysfunction at the 1985 and 1988 follow-up assessments, as part of the Yale Health and Aging Survey. Controlling for eighteen sociodemographic, behavioral, and biomedical variables using logistic regression, researchers reported that religious attendance in 1982 predicted less cognitive dysfunction in 1985, independent of other variables, but did not predict cognitive dysfunction in 1988. Lack of an effect in 1988, however, may have been due to high mortality among those with poor cognitive function and low religious attendance, since the sample size dropped by nearly one-third from 1,847 subjects in 1985 to 1,245 subjects in 1988.

Next, Canadian researchers presented research at the 2005 American Academy of Neurology meeting suggesting that religious involvement may delay or slow the progression of cognitive impairment in patients with Alzheimer's disease.[19] Kaufman and Freedman from Baycrest Centre for Geriatric Care in Toronto, Canada, used two measures of religion and spirituality, one with five items assessing religious attendance, private religious practices, and intrinsic religiosity, and one item asking participants to rate how religious or spiritual they were. Subjects were sixty-eight patients with Alzheimer's disease (average age seventy-eight), most with mild cases of the disease. They were from a mix of ethnic and religious backgrounds, including Christians, Jews, a Buddhist, and an atheist. Higher levels of self-rated spirituality and private religious activities were associated with a slower progression of Alzheimer's disease during the three-year follow-up period.

Not long after that, Hill and colleagues from the University of Texas reported the effects of religious attendance on cognitive functioning over six years in a large sample of older Hispanics.[20] Participants were involved in the Hispanic EPESE, an NIH-supported study that surveyed 3,050 older Mexican Americans (see chapter 7). After the baseline survey in 1993–1994, subjects were followed up in 1995–1996, 1998–1999, and 2000–2001. Cognitive functioning was assessed at each follow-up evaluation, and linear growth curve models were used to predict the effects of baseline religious attendance on cognitive function over time. Control variables included functional disability, sensory impairments, health behaviors, psychological distress, chronic diseases, and sociodemographic factors (age, gender, education, English proficiency, and social engagement). Investigators found that religious attendance predicted cognitive functioning in a dose-response manner. Those who attended religious services more than weekly (compared to nonattendees) declined more slowly in cognitive functioning by 0.75 points on the Mini-Mental State Exam per two-year period, or 2.25 points over the entire study period. For both weekly and more-than-weekly attendance, effects were significant.

Finally, Yeager and colleagues also found that religious

attendance was inversely related to cognitive impairment, even after controlling for baseline impairment, physical health, social factors, and health behaviors, in their sample of 2,930 older adults in Taiwan followed over four years.[21] These studies, all reported since 2003, suggest an important but poorly understood relationship between religious involvement and the development of cognitive impairment in later life.

## DIABETES

The development and course of diabetes is influenced by psychological factors, as noted in chapter 3, particularly by depression.[22] Thus, it is not surprising that diabetes—especially adult-onset (Type II) diabetes—may be related in some way to religious or spiritual beliefs. Although the research in this area remains in its infancy, a few studies report some interesting findings.

Van Olphen and colleagues studied a random sample of 679 African American women living on the east side of Detroit to assess the associations between religious involvement and health status.[23] Multivariate analyses controlling for education, age, income, marital status, living situation, and physical functioning found that respondents who "prayed more" experienced fewer depressive symptoms but more diabetes/hypertension. Those who "attended church more" had both fewer depressive symptoms and less diabetes/hypertension, with church-related social support partly explaining these associations. Since this was a cross-sectional study, however, we do not know whether the praying led to greater diabetes or patients sought support to cope with diabetes by turning to prayer. We also don't know whether frequent religious attendance led to less diabetes or whether their diabetic condition caused less church attendance.

More recently, Newlin surveyed 109 African American women with Type II diabetes, examining the relationship between spiritual well-being and diabetic control.[24] Spiritual well-being was measured using Palouzian and Ellison's Spiritual Well-Being Scale, which is composed of two ten-item subscales, a Religious Well-Being Scale and an Existential Well-Being Scale. HbA1c (a standard measure of diabetic control) was the primary outcome measure in this study. Subjects were dichotomized into those whose diabetic condition was controlled or approaching control and those who were uncontrolled. Results indicated that religious well-being significantly *increased* the odds of poor control, whereas existential well-being significantly *decreased* the odds of poor control, adjusting for demographic, clinical, and psychosocial factors. In this study, then, it was the more existential aspects of spiritual well-being that seemed to convey more benefits than the religious elements, although these aspects of spiritual well-being were highly correlated and this was again a cross-sectional study.

Religious involvement may also affect risk factors for development of diabetic complications. For example, King and colleagues analyzed data from the NHANES-III study (the most reputable regular survey of cardiovascular risk in the United States), looking at a sample of Americans over age forty that included 556 persons with diabetes.[25] The outcome of interest was the presence of elevated C-reactive protein. Recall that C-reactive protein levels strongly predict the development and course of heart disease, a common complication of diabetes. Investigators found that nonattendance at religious services was associated with more than twice the odds of having high C-reactive protein levels, compared to those for attendees. After adjusting for demographic variables, health status, smoking, social support, mobility, and body mass index, the association between religious attendance and C-reactive protein remained statistically significant. Since this was a cross-sectional study, investigators could not determine whether lack of religious involvement caused the increase in C-reactive protein levels. However, the findings might help to explain why lack of religious involvement in diabetics could be a factor in the future development of coronary artery disease.

Newlin and colleagues also found significant relationships between spiritual well-being (measured again using Palouzian and Ellison's Scale) and blood pressure in another study of twenty-two African American women with diabetes.[26] Although there was no relationship with diabetic control in this small study that lacked statistical power, total spiritual well-being and the religious well-being subscale were both significantly and inversely correlated with diastolic blood pressure. Thus, the finding of lower C-reactive protein and lower blood pressure among diabetics who are more religiously involved suggests that such involvement may reduce the risk of secondary complications in diabetes. Studies that directly examine relationships between religious involvement and diabetic complications, however, are yet to be done.

Religious beliefs may not always reduce the risk of diabetes or improve diabetic control. For example, researchers examined the relationship between diabetic control and religious beliefs in 106 Muslim men living in Leeds, England.[27] Results revealed that a large percentage of the sample were not controlling or managing their diabetes, including many men who were overweight. The general attitude among these men was to simply enjoy life and "leave the rest to Allah." Other cultural factors (such as greater weight and marriage traditions involving first cousins being more culturally acceptable) also played a role in poor diabetic control.

## CANCER

Many, many studies report that religious activities are related to better coping and greater quality of life among patients with cancer.[28] However, there is not a great deal of research on the impact of religious involvement on the development or course of malignant disorders.

It is well known that certain religious groups, such as Seventh-day Adventists, Mormons, the Amish, and others with strong taboos against drinking alcohol, smoking cigarettes, and other negative health behaviors, have lower rates of cancer.[29] Although these findings have been attributed primarily to diet and lifestyle, religious involvement may actually be additive to those of healthy lifestyles in reducing the risk of cancer mortality. For example, Enstrom used thirteen-year prospective data from the Alameda County Study (see chapter 7) to compare non-Mormons with healthy lifestyles with actively religious Mormons.[30] Among 2,290 whites of all religious faiths, the standard mortality rate from cancer was eighty-nine for the entire cohort, fifty-two for those who attended religious services at least weekly and didn't smoke, and thirteen for those who attended at least weekly and engaged in three health-related lifestyle practices (didn't smoke, exercised regularly, and got seven to eight hours of sleep a night). The standard mortality rates from cancer in this last group were even lower than in Mormon high priests who adhered to these three healthy lifestyle practices.

In a study of 253 patients with cancer from the Department of Oncology at a university hospital in Trondheim (Norway), Ringdal and colleagues reported the effects of baseline religiosity on survival over three years. Religiosity was assessed based on belief in God and extent to which religious beliefs provided support since the diagnosis of cancer. Religiousness was related to greater life satisfaction and to fewer feelings of hopelessness. When religiosity was included in a Cox regression analysis with hopelessness and life satisfaction, along with age, gender, cancer type, and physical functioning, the relative risk of dying for those with greater religiousness was 0.89. Removing hopelessness and life satisfaction from the model, decreased the relative risk of dying for those who were more religious to 0.86. Greater religiousness, then, predicted a 14 percent lower risk of dying, an effect that approached statistical significance ($p = 0.06$).[31]

Oman and colleagues examined the association between religious attendance and cancer mortality in a cohort of 6,545 persons followed for thirty-one years.[32] Less-frequent religious attendance (less than weekly) was associated with a greater risk of dying from cancer, after controlling for age, gender, ethnicity, birthplace, education, income, and non-Western religion. Adding initial health status as a control variable (number of chronic diseases, physical functioning, self-rated health, number of sick days in bed, and depression), however, reduced the association to nonsignificance. Including depression as a confounder along with measures of physical health status in this analysis could have explained why the effect lost statistical significance. Infrequent attendees, however, remained at greater risk of death from gastrointestinal cancer even after controlling for sociodemographic factors, and physical and mental health status. The latter risk was reduced to nonsignificance only after social factors and health behaviors were added to the model (i.e., factors that likely explained or mediated the effect of religion).

There is also evidence from Australia that greater religiousness may protect against the development of colorectal cancer. Kune and colleagues conducted a case-control study of 715 patients with colorectal cancer, whom they matched by age and sex with 727 community controls without cancer.[33] This was part of a population-based study of colorectal cancer incidence, etiology, and survival, titled the "Melbourne Colorectal Cancer Study." After a question about religious affiliation, subjects were asked, "Turning now to how religious you are, people may be described as not at all religious, slightly religious, moderately religious, or very religious. Which of these best describes you during your adult life?" Responses were divided into two groups for analysis—those that said they were not at all or only slightly religious versus those who were moderately or very religious. Subjects were then followed for five years. Results indicated that the religious group had a significantly lower relative risk of colorectal cancer (30 percent lower) than the nonreligious group. This association remained significant after controlling for other risk factors for colorectal cancer found in the Melbourne Colorectal Cancer Study, including family history of colorectal cancer, dietary risk factors, beer consumption, number of children, and, fro women, age at birth of the first child. Greater religiousness was also associated with a longer median survival time of sixty-two months, compared with fifty-two months for those who were not at all or minimally religious, although this difference was not statistically significant.

Finally, in a nine-year follow-up of 21,204 U.S. adults, Hummer and colleagues found that those who never attended religious services at baseline tended to have a greater risk of dying from cancer than those attending more than once per week, although this effect was explained by better health behaviors among the more religious.[34]

In general, associations between religiousness and cancer are not as strong as those between religion and cardiovascular disease. This is probably because cardiovascular disorders are more strongly influenced by psychosocial stress than is cancer (which probably has stronger genetic and environmental causes).[35] Bear in mind, however, that a reduction in the strength of the association between religious involvement and cancer mortality when health behaviors are controlled does not mean that there is no relationship between the two. Rather, it simply means that protection from cancer could be the result of better health behaviors by religious persons (who don't drink or smoke as much, engage in less risky sexual behaviors, etc.). Better health behaviors—just as good mental health and greater social support—are *explanatory* variables, not *confounding* variables in these relationships. I will discuss the differences between confounders and explanatory variables further in the next chapter.

## CONCLUSIONS

There is little doubt that religious involvement can help a person cope with the psychological and social stresses caused by heart disease, metabolic disorders like diabetes, cognitive changes with aging, and cancer. We know that these medical conditions are adversely affected by stress and negative emotions, factors that religious beliefs and activity may help to lessen or prevent. Therefore, it is not surprising that studies find fewer stress-related diseases or better disease outcomes among those who are more religious. While not all studies find such associations, many do, particularly when explanatory variables are distinguished from confounding variables in the statistical analyses. There is little or no evidence that religious involvement worsens stress-related diseases, although failure to seek medical attention early in the course of cardiovascular, metabolic, or malignant disorders (or the avoidance of medical care entirely) is likely to result in worse physical outcomes.[36] Religious involvement and medical care can work beautifully together. But when one or the other is excluded, patient outcomes will probably suffer.

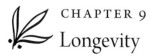

CHAPTER 9

# Longevity

NOTHING PROVIDES AS objective a measure of health as longevity—the length of our lifespans. People were particularly interested in Mrs. Harris because she lived beyond one hundred years. Everyone wanted to know how she accomplished this. Today, genetic factors have become a common explanation for many diseases. But genetics still has its limits, especially in helping us understand what causes a long, healthy life. Research shows that only a quarter of the lifespan (at most) can be attributed to genetic causes, and genes hardly influence longevity at all until after the age of sixty.[1] Even that contribution is disputed. For example, some researchers say that parental longevity has little association with the lifespan of offspring.[2] According to James W. Vaupel, director of the Laboratory of Survival and Longevity at the Max Planck Institute for Demographic Research in Rostock, Germany, how long a person's parents lived explains only about 3 percent of his or her lifespan.[3] Besides age and access to health care, other factors that could play a role are psychological, social, and behavioral.

The leading causes of death in the United States and around the world are heart disease, cancer, cerebrovascular disorders (including stroke), and infectious diseases (in that order).[4] It is clear from chapters 3 and 4 that these medical problems are directly affected by negative emotions, psychological and social stress, and poor health behaviors, as well as by genetic influences. Anything that improves coping with stress, that reduces negative emotions, and that encourages positive health behaviors should influence death rates from these diseases and affect overall mortality. One of these factors may be religious belief and practice.

## CONFOUNDERS VERSUS EXPLANATORY VARIABLES

Before proceeding further, I want to address an important point about which there is much confusion. I have already referred to this in previous chapters but would like now to explain this issue more fully. When analyzing the effects of a behavior such as religious attendance on mortality (or any health outcome), it is important to take into account factors likely to be associated with both religious attendance and survival. We know, on the one hand, that women are more likely than men both to attend religious services frequently and to live longer. We also know that frequent attendance is associated with higher education, which also predicts greater longevity. Likewise, people who are physically healthy without mobility problems are both more able to attend religious services and likely to live longer. On the other hand, members of minority groups (African Americans, Mexican Americans, etc.) tend to be more religiously involved than Caucasians and yet also have higher mortality rates. Likewise, people who are older tend to be more religious than those who are younger, and old age is certainly related to greater mortality. Thus, characteristics such as gender, education, ethnicity, age, and baseline physical mobility are called "confounders" because they may create the *false* impression that religious attendance is associated with either higher or lower mortality, when such correlations are simply due to the association between these other characteristics and longevity (religious attendance having nothing to do with it).

In contrast to confounders, there are other factors that help to explain how and why religious involvement might improve health and reduce mortality. As we discussed in chapter 4, the mechanism by which religious involvement is thought to affect physical health is through psychological, social, and behavioral pathways—i.e., by helping people cope with stress, increasing their social support, and encouraging healthier lifestyles and habits. These are called "explanatory" or "mediating variables," not confounders. In other words, these factors help to explain how religion affects health; they do not create false associations that have nothing to do with religion, as confounders do.

I will now illustrate how failure to distinguish confounders from explanatory factors can result in inaccurate interpretations of research data. Let us consider a meteorologist who is studying the effects of hurricanes on the frequency of automobile accidents in the Caribbean islands. One factor related to both motor-vehicle accidents and hurricanes is the time of year. In summer, there are many who vacation in Caribbean islands and the result is more accidents as a consequence of more people on the road. Coincidentally, there are also more hurricanes at this time of the year. Therefore, if a researcher finds an association between hurricanes and accidents, he or she may falsely conclude that hurricanes cause automobile accidents. To avoid this, he or she must take into account "time of the year" (a confounder) in the statistical analyses.

On the other hand, we know that hurricanes probably do indeed cause accidents because of the tremendous wind and rain that they produce. Here, the wind and rain caused by the hurricane are called explanatory variables. They explain how the hurricane causes accidents. However, if the researcher "controlled" for the wind and the rain in her analysis (considering them confounders, rather than explanatory variables), then the association between hurricanes and accidents would disappear, and she might falsely conclude that there is no real relationship between hurricanes and accidents.

Distinguishing confounders from explanatory factors is extremely important when studying, analyzing, and interpreting relationships found between religiosity and mortality. If the association found between religious involvement and mortality disappears when confounders are controlled for, then there is truly no relationship between the two. If a relationship remains between religion and mortality after confounders are controlled, however, then that relationship is a real one. Many investigators, particularly the critics of the religion–health relationship, often fail to distinguish between confounders and explanatory variables. They lump explanatory variables into the same category as confounders and interpret the results similarly—i.e., that if the relationship between religion and health weakens to nonsignificance after controlling for all characteristics (including explanatory variables), then there is really no relationship between religion and health. Such a conclusion, however, is simply false.

Critics counter my argument above by saying that there is no way to prove that religious involvement actually leads to or causes greater social support, better mental health, or better health behaviors and that these cannot be established as explanatory variables until such proof exists.[5] They say that, perhaps because of personality or genetic factors, religiously active people are simply more social or more mentally fit or make better decisions about health habits and health behaviors. Only randomized controlled trials (RCTs), critics say, can resolve this issue (i.e., subjects are randomized either to a religious intervention or a control group, and social support, mental health, and health behavior outcomes are measured over time).

There is ample epidemiological evidence, however, that religious involvement does predict future increases in social support, faster resolution of depression, and greater reduction in smoking or heavy alcohol consumption.[6] Such epidemiological evidence can come very close to establishing causation, as described by Hill over three decades ago.[7] Furthermore, there are a number of RCTs that show religious interventions for depression and anxiety result in faster remission of symptoms than secular therapies or no treatment (see chapter 5). Thus, the weight of the evidence today favors psychological, social, and behavioral factors being categorized as explanatory variables or mediators of the religion–health relationship, not as confounders.

## RELIGIOUS INVOLVEMENT AND MORTALITY

In 2000, McCullough and colleagues conducted a meta-analysis of forty-two studies with a total of 126,000 participants that examined the effects of religious involvement on survival.[8] Based on this meta-analysis, they concluded that religious involvement increased survival by 29 percent, after controlling for both confounders *and explanatory variables* (if anything, this report underestimated the effects because researchers controlled for explanatory variables in addition to confounders). Sensitivity analysis indicated that it would take 1,418 studies showing no effect to overturn the observed pattern of results. The effects were stronger in women than in men and were greatest for attendance at religious services (versus private religious activities).

For attendance, there were twenty-one studies involving 107,910 participants. In these models, weekly religious attendance was associated with a 37 percent increased survival. That odds ratio is consistent with results from the four largest, most-recent, and best-designed studies of the attendance–survival relationship, even after controlling both for confounders (age, gender, race, etc.) *and* explanatory variables (mental health, social support, health behaviors, etc.).[9] This finding is also consistent with a conservative review of the studies by an independent panel of experienced researchers who reported an increased likelihood of survival ranging from 33 percent to 42 percent (depending on whether both confounders and explanatory variables or only confounders were controlled for).[10]

Controlling for both confounders and explanatory variables in such models reduces the association between religious attendance and longevity, with some critics concluding that either there is no relationship or the relationship is weak and insignificant. The real strength of the relationship between religious involvement and mortality, however, is the one that results when only confounders are controlled for. Explanatory variables should then be entered into statistical models to determine which of these factors explain or mediate the relationship and how much of the effect they explain. Based on explanatory mechanisms discussed in chapter 4, we would actually *expect* the relationship between religious involvement and mortality to disappear completely when explanatory factors are taken fully into account. The fact that the relationship between attendance and lower mortality persists even after controlling for these factors remains a bit of a mystery. One might speculate, however, that it is because we are not yet able completely to measure and control for factors that explain how religion promotes longevity.

## Public-Health Impact

As we saw in McCullough's meta-analysis of forty-two studies (see note 8 in this chapter), the effect of religious attendance on survival is relatively small. Nevertheless, does it have significance from a public-health standpoint? To answer this question, it helps to compare the effects of other more-established medical and psychosocial treatments on mortality. This is what McCullough did when responding to critics of his meta-analysis.[11] For example, Jolliffe and colleagues conducted a meta-analysis on the effectiveness of comprehensive cardiac rehabilitation and exercise in patients with coronary artery disease.[12] Based on 7,683 participants in randomized controlled trials, they found that exercise by itself increased the likelihood of survival by 37 percent and that comprehensive cardiac rehabilitation increased survival by 15 percent.

Similarly, Smith and colleagues examined the impact of cholesterol-lowering drugs (such as Lipitor) on all-cause mortality among patients at high risk for coronary artery disease.[13] They reported that the odds of survival were increased by 35 percent for those receiving the medication. With regard to psychosocial treatments, Linden and colleagues conducted a meta-analysis of thirteen randomized controlled trials examining the effect on mortality of failure to receive psychosocial interventions following myocardial infarction.[14] This meta-analysis, which involved 1,745 participants, reported that those not receiving this intervention had a 70 percent increased likelihood of dying during the first two years of follow-up and a 35 percent increased likelihood after two years.

Of course, randomized clinical trials are quite different from observational, naturalistic studies of religious attendance. Comprehensive cardiac rehabilitation or psychosocial treatments following heart attacks, however, usually involve intensive physical, psychosocial, social, or drug treatments, which would be expected to yield relatively large effects. With regard to observational studies comparable to those examining the impact of religious attendance, Holman and colleagues examined the effects of hazardous alcohol use (two to four drinks per day for women and four to six drinks per day for men) and of harmful alcohol use (more than four drinks per day for women and more than six drinks per day for men) on mortality, based on sixteen observational studies.[15] Hazardous drinkers experienced a 24 percent increased risk of dying, while harmful drinkers experienced a 37 percent increased risk of dying.

Now we return to our earlier question: Does the McCullough meta-analysis of religion and mortality compare favorably with these aforementioned studies of more-established treatments and other factors that we know affect longevity? I would argue, along with McCullough, that they do fall into the same range. While such effects may appear small, they nevertheless have a large public-health impact. The result is that heavy alcohol use is widely discouraged and the treatments for coronary artery disease described above are now a standard part of medical care.

Other methods have also been used to place into perspective the effect that religious attendance has on mortality. Using age-specific, actuarial death rates modified by odds ratios obtained from meta-analyses like those above, Hall examined the impact of weekly religious attendance on years of additional life, compared with regular physical exercise and use of cholesterol-lowering drugs.[16] He found that weekly religious attendance conferred an additional two to three years of life compared to three to five years of life from regular physical exercise and 2.5 years to 3.5 years of life for cholesterol-lowering drugs. He calculated that the approximate cost per life-year gained was between $2,000 and $6,000 for regular exercise, $3,000 to $10,000 for weekly religious attendance, and $4,000 to $14,000 for cholesterol-lowering drugs. The article, published in a peer-reviewed medical journal, was provocatively titled, "Religious Attendance: More Cost-Effective Than Lipitor?"

If regular religious attendance has an influence on reducing mortality comparable to that of cholesterol-lowering drugs, regular exercise, avoidance of hazardous or harmful alcohol intake, psychosocial interventions after a heart attack, or comprehensive cardiac rehabilitation, then the impact that religious involvement might have on public health is substantial. Add to this the fact that well over one-hundred-million people in the United States attend religious services at least weekly, the effect that such involvement may have on the overall health of the population is huge.

Because the relationships between religious involvement and longevity are based on observational studies, not randomized clinical trials, it is not possible to prove beyond a shadow of a doubt that religious involvement actually leads to greater longevity. Unidentified confounders may always exist that are related to both religious involvement and longevity, and, if these were measured and controlled for, then perhaps the relationship with longevity would disappear. The only way to resolve this dilemma is to randomize people either to religious involvement or no religious involvement and then follow them to their death. However, one would have to ensure that, over time, those randomized to the religious group stay religious and those randomized to the control group stay nonreligious. This, however, would be an unfeasible and certainly unethical experiment, since you can't force people to stay religious or prevent them from becoming religious. Most epidemiological data on characteristics and behaviors related to longevity (cigarette smoking, for example) suffer from this limitation. At some point, however, the evidence becomes so consistent, widespread, and in line with theoretical expectations that causal inferences can be made with reasonable confidence (see Hill's criteria for causality, note 7 in this chapter). I think the evidence is approaching this level for religious attendance.

## THE BEST STUDIES

While useful, meta-analyses tend to average out the findings from all studies, regardless of whether their methodological design and execution were done well or poorly. A poorly designed and executed study is less likely to uncover an effect (or reveal the true magnitude of the association) than a well-done study. For that reason, I will review some of the best religion–mortality studies below to give the reader a sense of what some of this research has found.

### Alameda County Study

Researchers at the Human Population Laboratory in Berkeley, California, examined the effects of religious attendance on mortality over twenty-eight years. Strawbridge and colleagues reported their findings in the *American Journal of Public Health* in 1997.[17] Complete data on religious involvement, confounders, explanatory variables, and vital status (mortality) were available on 5,286 of the original 6,928 participants (see chapter 7). In 1965 when the study began, 25.1 percent of the sample attended religious services weekly or more often. Frequent attendees were more likely to be women and African Americans, had more social connections, were less likely to smoke cigarettes, were less likely to be heavy drinkers, were more likely to be overweight, and were *more likely* to have limitations in their physical mobility. Among those with mobility limitations, the percentage attending religious services at least weekly was 35.3 percent, compared to 24.8 percent for those who were physically healthy and without such physical restrictions. This last finding is particularly important because most critics complain that frequent church attendees have greater mobility at the start of the study than less-frequent attendees, and that those who are less mobile are less likely to go to church and more likely to die because of underlying health problems. In this study, the opposite was true!

In determining the effects of religious attendance in 1965 on mortality status in 1994, investigators not only controlled for characteristics of participants in 1965 but also assessed those characteristics throughout the twenty-eight-year follow-up (called "time-dependent covariates"), enabling them to take into account statistically the changes in those characteristics over time. Controlling for confounders such as age, gender, ethnicity, and education, the analyses showed that those who attended religious services at least weekly in 1965 were 36 percent less likely than less-frequent attendees to be dead when followed up in 1994. Controlling further for health conditions (including the explanatory variable mental health, i.e., how depressed they were) and mobility restrictions reduced the effect from 36 percent to 33 percent. Controlling further for social connections (an explanatory variable) reduced it to 31 percent, and, finally, controlling for health practices (an explanatory variable) reduced the effect to 23 percent.

The effects of religious attendance were greatest in women. The impact of weekly attendance in women (a 37 percent reduction in mortality) approximated the effect of having never smoked cigarettes (47 percent reduction in mortality).[18] Does that have any practical significance? You bet it does.

These investigators also examined the mechanism by which religious attendance might have affected survival. During the twenty-eight-year follow-up, they found that frequent attendees were 90 percent more likely to stop smoking, 38 percent more likely to increase exercising, 79 percent more likely to stay married, 58 percent more likely to increase nonchurch community memberships, and 50 percent more likely to increase number of close friends/relatives seen each month (see note 17). In a later report by Strawbridge and colleagues, they found that frequent attendees in 1965 were nearly two-and-one-half times more likely to remit from depression, and women who were heavy drinkers in 1965 were almost five times more likely to stop drinking if they attended religious services at least weekly (all of these analyses controlled for age, gender, education, and self-rated health).[19]

These findings from one of the largest and most respected epidemiological studies ever conducted helps to counter the argument above by critics that psychological, social, and behavioral factors are not explanatory variables. This study provides evidence suggesting that religious involvement does indeed lead to improvements in these psychological, social, and health behavior characteristics over time.

### National Health Interview Survey

Hummer and colleagues from the Population Research Center at the University of Texas at Austin examined data on religious attendance and mortality from a random national sample of 21,204 adults followed from 1987 to 1995.[20] Persons who never attended religious services were 87 percent more likely to die during follow-up versus those attending more than once a week, controlling for age, gender, ethnicity, and region of the country (what we would call confounders). This translated into a seven-year difference in survival after age twenty. Among African Americans, the difference in life expectancy between nonattendees and more-than-weekly attendees was fourteen years. African Americans who never attended religious services lived to an average age of 66.4 years, compared to 80.1 years for those who attended services more than once per week.

After controlling for education, income, activity limitations, self-reported health, and days spent in bed, the effect was reduced to 72 percent. Controlling further for explanatory or mediating variables (social factors and health behaviors) reduced the effect to 50 percent (still highly statistically significant). Causes of death for which effects of religious attendance were strongest were circulatory diseases (heart, stroke, etc.), respiratory diseases, diabetes, infectious diseases, and external causes (such as accidents). A weak relationship with cancer disappeared when confounders were taken into account.

## Established Populations for Epidemiological Studies in the Elderly (EPESE)

In response to the Alameda County Study on the West Coast, my colleagues and I decided to examine the relationship between religious attendance and longevity among older adults on the East coast.[21] Information on religious attendance and many of the other variables measured in the Alameda County Study were available on four thousand randomly selected persons age sixty-five or older who participated in the North Carolina site of the NIH-supported EPESE (see chapter 6). Although our follow-up time was shorter (1986–92) and our population was older, we anticipated that the effects of regular attendance might be more evident in this population that was experiencing health problems related to aging.

We created similar statistical models as the Alameda County Study, including demographics (age, gender, education, ethnicity), physical health (physical function, chronic conditions, self-rated health) and mental health (depression, stressful life events), social connections (marital status, social network, supportive confidantes, satisfaction with support, and support received), and health practices (smoking, alcohol, weight). Before control variables (confounders) were taken into account, subjects who attended religious services at least weekly were 46 percent less likely to die during the follow-up period. Including demographic confounders in the model reduced the effect from 46 percent to 41 percent; including physical and mental health in the model (a combination of confounders and explanatory variables) reduced the effect to 31 percent; and including social connections and health behaviors (both explanatory variables) reduced the effect to 28 percent. Thus, even after considering both potential confounders of the relationship and factors that might explain how religious attendance reduces mortality, there remained a significant and substantial effect. As in the Alameda County Study, the effect in our study was strongest among women (35 percent reduction versus 17 percent reduction in men) but was significant statistically for both genders in all models.

### Studies outside the United States

In the only published study to date from Europe (to my knowledge), the effects of religious characteristics on mortality were examined in a sample of 734 community dwellers over age seventy living in Glostrup, Denmark.[22] Religious characteristics were measured at baseline, and subjects were then followed for twenty years, collecting mortality data. Those who indicated that religious affiliation was meaningful (versus not) experienced a 30 percent lower risk of dying. Those who attended religious services often or rarely (versus never) experienced a 27 percent reduced risk of dying. No relationship was found for watching religious media. When gender and education were controlled, the effect of affiliation was reduced to nonsignificance in men but persisted in women. When physical health and mental health were controlled, the effect for affiliation in women lost significance (although some of this may have been due to mediation, not confounding). For religious attendance, the effect weakened when gender and education were controlled but remained significant, particularly among women. When physical and mental health variables were controlled, the effect persisted, reflecting a 22 percent reduction in mortality for churchgoers. When explanatory factors such as social support and health behaviors were controlled (mediators), the effect weakened further but remained statistically significant.

In the only study published to date from Asia (to my knowledge), Yeager and colleagues examined relationships between religious attendance and mortality rates over four years in a sample of 3,800 persons in Taiwan, China.[23] Frequency of religious attendance was inversely related to mortality, an effect that showed a gradient, with those attending "often" having lower mortality than those attending "sometimes," compared to those attending "never." As noted earlier, this study is of particular interest since over 92 percent of the sample was non-Christian (primarily Buddhist, Taoist, or traditional). As in other studies, effects persisted after controlling for confounders and explanatory variables.

## PRAYER, LONGEVITY, AND HEALTH

Besides religious attendance, a few studies have examined the relationship between prayer or meditation and survival.[24] In a clinical trial that examined the effects of Transcendental Meditation, Alexander and colleagues at Maharishi University randomly assigned seventy-three retired persons (mean age eighty-one years) to groups practicing (a) Transcendental Meditation (a Hindu-based prayer practice), (b) Mindfulness Meditation (a Buddhist prayer practice), (c) mental relaxation, or (d) no treatment control.[25] After three years, 100 percent of the Transcendental Meditation patients were alive, compared to 88 percent of the Mindfulness Meditation group, 65 percent of the mental-relaxation group, and 77 percent of the no-treatment controls.

In a two-year prospective study of 444 hospitalized patients, Pargament and colleagues examined the effects of frequency of prayer, meditation, or Bible study on mortality. No effect of prayer on mortality was found. Yeager and colleagues studying the Eastern religious sample described earlier also found no effect for prayer on mortality.[26]

The difficulty in examining prayer is that, as people become sicker and nearer to death, they begin to pray more. This is exactly the opposite problem that occurs with religious attendance, where, as people get sicker, they are less able to attend religious services. Because many turn to prayer as their health worsens, this may create an artificial positive association between prayer and mortality that could conceal or neutralize any protective effects when statistical analyses are done. In the EPESE study described above, my colleagues and I at Duke attempted to get around this problem by dividing the sample at baseline into two groups based on level of disability: (1) 2,058 older adults with at least one impairment of "activities of daily living" versus (2) 1,793 subjects with no physical impairments (prayer frequency was available on 3,851 of 4,000 subjects).[27] We then examined the effects of prayer frequency on mortality separately in each group, hypothesizing that the effects of prayer on mortality would be more evident over time in the healthy group because turning to religion in response to health problems would be less of an issue.

That is exactly what we found. After controlling for confounders, no effect of prayer on survival was found among the 2,058 subjects who were already suffering from disabilities. Among the 1,793 healthy subjects, however, those who prayed were 73 percent more likely to survive during follow-up compared to those who did not pray. When demographics (confounders) were controlled, the effect was reduced to 66 percent. When health variables (including the explanatory variables depression and stressful life events) were added to the model, the effect was reduced a bit further to 63 percent. Therefore, at a minimum, after controlling for confounders, those who prayed were 63 percent more likely to survive than those who did not pray. Controlling further for social connections and health behaviors (both explanatory variables) reduced the effect to 55 percent. Thus, healthy subjects who prayed were nearly two-thirds more likely to survive, and only a small percentage of this effect could be explained on the basis of mental, social, or behavioral factors.

Although I could not locate any more recent studies on prayer and mortality, several studies have examined effects of prayer on health outcomes or functioning. As described earlier, Ai and colleagues examined the effects of religious coping and prayer on postoperative global functioning after cardiac surgery in 335 patients.[28] Regression analyses revealed that postoperative prayer frequency was associated with worse postoperative functioning in the *cross-sectional* analysis, although the investigators acknowledged that this may have reflected a turning to prayer as a result of poorer functioning. In another study, Contrada and colleagues at Rutgers examined the effects of religiousness on complications experienced during recovery from heart surgery.[29] A single question assessing frequency of private prayer in 142 patients one week prior to surgery. Frequency of prayer did not predict either complications or length of hospital stay, although analyses were not stratified by baseline health status as we did in the EPESE study above.

Finally, in one of the few clinical trials of on-site, *in-person* intercessory prayer on health outcomes, Matthews and colleagues assigned forty patients with class II or III rheumatoid arthritis to either a prayer intervention or a wait-list control group.[30] The prayer intervention, conducted over three days, consisted of six hours of education and six hours of hands-on prayer by others. Outcomes examined were measures of arthritis severity assessed at three-month intervals for one year. Researchers found that patients receiving hands-on direct contact prayer showed significantly greater improvement in pain and joint function during follow-up.

## RELIGION AND GREATER MORTALITY

Although most studies show either beneficial effects of religious involvement on mortality or no effect, at least one study has found that religious struggles (also called negative religious coping) were associated with greater mortality over time. My colleagues and I followed 444 hospitalized patients (age fifty-five plus) for an average of two years, examining the impact of religious struggle during hospitalization on survival.[31] Religious struggle or conflict was assessed using a seven-item scale that captured patients' feelings that God was punishing or had abandoned them, that they were abandoned by their faith community, that God did not have the power to make a difference, and other negative religious thoughts (zero to three ratings on agreement, with total scores ranging from zero to twenty-one). After controlling for demographic, physical health, and mental and social factors, higher religious-struggle scores predicted a greater risk of mortality over time. For every one-point increase on the religious-struggles scale, there was a 6 percent increase in mortality. Two of the seven religious-struggles questions ("Wondered whether God had abandoned me" and "Questioned God's love for me") increased risk of mortality by 28 percent and 22 percent, respectively.

## Conclusions

Religious involvement, particularly attending religious services, is associated with a lower risk of mortality based on reports following subjects for up to three decades. These studies involved random regional and national samples in the United States and outside the United States in Europe and Asia. They have included Christians (predominantly) and non-Christians. Effects on mortality have also been observed for prayer and meditation but primarily in those without health problems. Religious struggles, however, predict greater mortality. These findings suggest that religious involvement is generally associated with lower mortality, particularly when religious beliefs are without conflict.

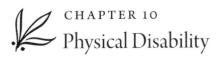

CHAPTER 10

# Physical Disability

AN ALARMING PICTURE emerges when we consider that people are living longer—an unprecedented number will likely spend many of their later years with physical disabilities. This challenge demands innovative responses, and these may include religion or spirituality.

Reducing the physical disability that occurs naturally with age, that results from disease, or that comes after acute injury is likely to be a high priority for health-care systems both inside and outside the United States during the twenty-first century. Besides being immensely costly, physical disability also has psychological consequences that can worsen disability and send a person into a downward spiral of increasing dependency and decreasing motivation to do anything about it.

Physical disability is a threat to our independence and sense of control, especially in Western cultures. Not being able to care for one's own physical needs, for whatever reason, can produce great suffering and distress. Dependency on others can adversely affect a person's self-esteem and sense of purpose and meaning in life. Measures of physical disability are related to greater rates of depression and other negative emotions in almost every study in which this has been examined.[1] Even among older adults, when disability may be considered "on time" with regard to age, 40 percent of those with disability admit to experiencing emotional distress whenever they need to be helped.[2] That percentage is likely to increase even higher in younger adults with chronic disabilities, where such disabilities are not "on time."

Once again, here is an area where religion might make a difference. In patients with chronic medical illness or disability, a host of studies shows that religious involvement is a frequently used coping behavior. Those who cope using religion have lower rates of depression and faster recovery from depression (see chapter 5). There is also evidence that those with health problems and disability more often turn to religion for strength and comfort than do persons without health problems.[3] Again, this widespread "turning to religion" in response to disability complicates statistical analyses that seek to examine the impact of religious involvement (particularly private religious activities and importance of religion) on the development of disability. This problem is similar to that encountered when researchers try to examine the relationship between prayer and mortality, since so many persons suddenly start praying—or at least pray a lot more—when they become sick.

Causes of physical disability are important when considering the possible effects that religious involvement might have. After infections and parasitic diseases, the worldwide leading cause of disability (defined as years of life living with disability) is not a physical health problem at all—it's *major depression*, which affects over 50 million people worldwide.[4] Not only does depression cause disability, but it is also a consequence of disability. Inability to cope with the changes, losses, and restrictions brought on by physical illness frequently results in depression. As patients become more and more depressed, they have less and less motivation to rehabilitate and become less fully engaged in their own recovery. The depressed person feels tired all the time, can't concentrate, and often doesn't feel motivated to make the effort necessary to get better. Life begins to lose meaning, and there seems little hope that anything they do will make any difference. Some become so discouraged that they seek to stop this endless torture by hastening their own death, either through noncompliance with medical treatments or by taking more direct measures. Thus, anything that helps to prevent depression or accelerate its resolution will likely affect a person's ability and desire to function mentally, socially, and physically.

## THEORETICAL CONSIDERATIONS

How might religious beliefs and activities influence the development or course of physical disability? Throughout this book, I have emphasized the importance of religion as a coping behavior. Therefore, it should not be surprising that, by helping patients to cope, religious beliefs and behaviors might help reduce the physical disability that results from depression and reduce the depression that results from disability. For example, involvement in religious community activities results in the development of important social relationships, which may motivate individuals to get out of their homes and attend church-related social functions. Both the social support and the physical engagement that result from such activities may help to prevent the onset or worsening of disability. Religious beliefs, reinforced in social settings, may provide meaning and purpose despite the development of disability and dependency. In fact, religion may be *especially* helpful in such circumstances.

Religious involvement has been associated with increased morale, life satisfaction, and faster recovery from depression in numerous studies of older adults with chronic health problems (see chapter 5).[5] For example, in a study of 850 medically ill hospitalized older men, my colleagues and I found an inverse relationship between religious coping and depression. This relationship was particularly strong among those with more severe functional disability.[6] In a second study of older depressed patients of both genders followed for nearly one year, we found that the effect of religiosity on speeding remission from depression was particularly strong among those with persistent disability.[7] Likewise, in a study of elderly women recovering from surgery for hip fracture, greater religiousness predicted longer walking distances at the time of discharge.[8] As hope reappears and depression lifts, motivation increases and patients feel more like exercising and involving themselves in self-care types of activities that will ultimately slow the development of chronic disability or speed recovery from it.

## DISABILITY STUDIES AMONG THE ELDERLY

Several prospective studies have now reported that religious involvement, as expected, predicts slower progression of disability over time. In 1982, Idler and colleagues assessed 2,781 persons aged sixty-five years or older involved in the New Haven–Yale site of the Established Populations for Epidemiologic Studies in the Elderly (EPESE). They then followed this group for twelve years, measuring subsequent disability levels yearly from 1983 to 1988 and then finally in 1994.[9] Religious attendance measured in 1982 predicted significantly less disability in the following six years, from 1983 to 1988. Although the effect in 1994 failed to reach statistical significance, the effect size was similar in magnitude to that found in earlier years (but, by 1994, the sample size had dwindled from 2,088 initially down to only 830, reducing the statistical power to detect the difference). These effects were independent of baseline disability level, number of chronic conditions, medications, cognitive function, age, ethnicity, income, marital status, education, and gender. Subjective religiousness in that study, however, was unrelated to future disability levels after controlling for religious attendance.

Idler and colleagues also found that religious attendance had more of an impact on preventing physical disability than physical disability had on preventing religious attendance. This is a crucial point. It suggests that, while many older persons stop going to church in the short term because of increasing disability, even more retain their ability to function as a result of attending religious services. This helps to counter the argument by critics that religious attendance is related to mortality only because those who are closer to death are more physically disabled, which prevents them from going to church and confounds the relationship. The New Haven–Yale wing of the EPESE study suggests that, while disability may prevent religious attendance in the short term, religious attendance also prevents disability and that the latter effect is stronger and longer lasting than the former.

This may be particularly true for certain minority groups. For example, a study of over five hundred older African Americans (an ethnic group that is at particularly high risk for functional disability in later life) reported that health limitations did not prevent church attendance significantly.[10] The reason was that these persons often made extraordinary efforts to continue to attend services despite physical disability.[11] They often appeared at religious services using canes, walkers, or wheelchairs, whatever it took to get there.

The results of the New Haven–Yale study have been replicated in subsequent research. For example, comparing two waves of a national, longitudinal study of 4,071 older adults, Benjamins found a statistically significant relationship between religious-service attendance at baseline (weekly attendance or more) and lower levels of functional limitations five years later (1995 to 2000).[12] This association was independent of baseline functional limitations, demographics, socioeconomic status, physical health, social resources, mental health, and health behaviors (i.e., was independent of both confounders and explanatory factors).

Importance of religion (religious salience), however, was associated with *greater* disability (the opposite of that for religious attendance). The author provided no explanation for this unexpected finding, other than suggesting that further research was needed. However, it is likely that those with greater disability were more likely to turn to religion for comfort and report that it was important to them, interfering with the researcher's ability to show a positive effect for religious importance on forestalling disability.

In a recent study involving 784 randomly sampled older adults in central Alabama who were assessed and then followed for three years, Park and colleagues found that frequent religious attendance was associated with less functional disability (measured by ability to perform activities of daily living) at baseline.[13] Furthermore, frequent attendance predicted a slower rate of functional decline over time, an effect that persisted after controlling for age, race, gender, living arrangement, marital status, social support, informal support, income adequacy, education, comorbidity, and cognitive function.

As in the New Haven–Yale study, however, private religious activities and personal commitment (frequency of prayer and degree of intrinsic religiosity) were unrelated to physical functioning either at baseline or across the three-year follow-up. This lack of an effect could have been due to the high frequency of prayer and level of intrinsic religiosity in this rural, older sample in the center of the Bible Belt. Lack of variation in private religious activity and intensity of religious belief could have reduced the power of the statistical analyses to detect significant effects.

Not all studies, however, find that religious activity (even religious attendance) predicts slower functional decline. For example, Kelley-Moore and Ferraro found no relationship between baseline religious attendance and functional limitations three years later in a national sample of 1,282 adults over age sixty years (nor was there any effect for private religious activities or religious salience).[14] Although these investigators did not show an impact for religious attendance on preventing disability, they also did not show a sustained effect of disability on preventing religious attendance. While disability levels were inversely related to religious attendance in cross-sectional models, baseline functional disability did not predict future attendance years later, again suggesting, as Idler's study had, that disability affects religious attendance only in the short term and has little effect on long-term patterns of attendance.

Thus, while most studies show that religious involvement (particularly religious attendance) may prevent the onset and progression of disability, there is almost no evidence that disability prevents religious attendance over the long term. Disabled persons, particularly those from minority communities, make extraordinary efforts to keep on going to church—since that is where they find their support and hope.

## Fear of Falling

Using a different approach to studying the relationship between religion and disability, Reyes-Ortiz and colleagues examined the link between religious attendance and fear of falling—the fear of falling down and injuring oneself when walking—which is a known predecessor of physical disability in older adults.[15] The study involved a random sample of 1,341 noninstitutionalized Mexican Americans aged seventy-two and over. Subjects participating in the third wave of the Hispanic EPESE (see chapter 6) were asked about religious attendance and then were followed for two years when they were assessed for fear of falling. Results indicated that religious attendance significantly predicted less fear of falling independent of other baseline predictors. Other significant predictors of fear of falling controlled for in the analysis were female gender, poorer objective lower-body performance, history of previous falls, arthritis, hypertension, and urinary incontinence.

This finding is important because falls are the third most common cause of disability worldwide.[16] Fear of falling is known to be a strong predictor of worsening physical function, osteoporosis, and hip fracture in older adults. When elders develop fear of falling, they become afraid to get out of bed and stop exercising. This results in immobility, which, in turn, increases the risk of osteoporosis, muscle deconditioning, and problems with balance, so that, when they are forced to move about (often to use the commode at night), they fall, seriously injure themselves, and end up in a nursing home.[17] Since fear of falling is a strong predictor of age-related declines in physical health and since staying active in a religious community reduces that fear, this may be one reason why older adults who frequently attend religious services retain their physical functioning with age.

## PERCEPTIONS OF HEALTH

Perceptions of health may also influence how older adults think of themselves and what they can do physically. In the previously cited Yale Health and Aging Project (see chapter 8), which included 1,617 women and 1,139 men surveyed in 1982, Idler examined the interaction between strength or comfort derived from religion, number of chronic conditions, and level of self-reported disability (based on impairments in activities of daily living).[18] She found that, for men who said that they received no comfort or strength from religion, any given level of chronic medical conditions was associated with greater perceived physical disability. In other words, men who said they received a great deal of comfort from religion reported less disability at any given level of chronic illness than did men who said they received no comfort from religion. This finding suggests that religious coping can modify the impact that chronic conditions have on level of perceived disability.

In a later paper, Idler examined further how self-perception can impact a person's physical functioning and how religion can influence that.[19] She interviewed 146 patients with various types of disabilities at an urban rehabilitation clinic, testing two seemly disparate hypotheses: (1) those with poorer health or greater disability are more likely to say that they have sought help from religion, and (2) persons with stronger religious senses of self-identity and better self-ratings of health will have a stronger nonphysical sense of self (which Idler defined as the sense of self derived from nonphysical characteristics, including religious or spiritual identities). That could help explain why persons who were more religious report less disability at any given degree of objective physical illness. Both of Idler's hypotheses were supported by the quantitative data she collected and the qualitative reports elicited from participants. She found that, as patients became sicker or more disabled, they derived greater comfort from religion, which, in turn, affected their self-perceptions of disability. Nonphysical sense of self, which depended partly on religious or spiritual factors, influenced perceptions of disability in such a way that those who were more religious saw themselves as more able and functional. That perception, then, influenced their behavior, which helped them to retain their ability to function.

## DISABILITY IN THE YOUNG

Much of the research I've discussed above is related to older adults and the development of chronic disability over time. Not nearly as much is known about the relationship between religion and disability in young persons affected by an accident or injury that leaves them dependent on others, possibly for the rest of their lives. When disability occurs suddenly and in the prime of life, the burden of coping and degree of loss perceived is much greater. Increasing disability in advanced age is to be expected. Not so, however, when a young person is paralyzed from the neck down after a diving accident or car wreck. Not so with the young, recently married man who has both legs blown off by a roadside bomb in Iraq. Not so for the young woman who has just been diagnosed with a progressive neurological condition that will leave her dependent for the rest of her life and may affect her plans to get married, have children, or pursue a career.

Qualitative studies of young persons with disabilities and their parents suggest that religious beliefs help to stabilize their lives, provide meaning, assist with coping, and convey other benefits as a result of being involved in a faith community.[20] Quantitative studies suggest that the quality of life and life satisfaction of persons with progressive neurological disorders such as amyotrophic lateral sclerosis (Lou Gehrig's disease) and spinal cord injuries depend not only on physical functioning but also on spiritual factors and social supports (which, in turn, have the ability to affect physical functioning).[21] However, these conclusions are based on small, cross-sectional studies. Little research has examined religious and spiritual factors over time as they relate to emotional, social, physical, and occupational outcomes in young persons experiencing sudden disabilities. To my knowledge, no studies at all have been done examining spiritual interventions. This area, then, is in great need of attention.

## Conclusions

Many patients turn to religion as a way of coping with the disability and dysfunction caused by chronic medical illness. Religion is also effective for coping with the depression that grows out of disability. Religious involvement may also affect the development and course of physical disability because of religion's impact on mental health, social health, sense of self, and perceived ability to function. The best evidence for this comes from studies examining the effects of religious attendance on physical disability over time in older populations. Religious involvement may also help lessen the fears and self-doubts that prevent older people from walking, getting out, and participating with others in social activities.

Still unclear, however, is the reason why private religious involvement does not predict a slowing in the development of disability. One reason may be that people increasingly turn to religion as disability worsens—so it incorrectly appears as if religion has no impact on slowing down disability. Either way, further research is needed to understand better this dynamic of the interactions between changing religiousness and changing disability over time. Another large research gap is in the study of young persons with spinal cord injuries, amputations, and other injuries from accidents, war, or disease, who suffer from long-term disability. Religious involvement may be a resource to help these young persons to live more meaningful and productive lives, although whether this is true or to what extent remains unknown.

## CHAPTER 11

# Clinical Applications

BASED ON THE RESEARCH presented in previous chapters, health professionals should readily see how a person's religious faith may influence his or her health, coping with illness, and medical decisions. What can a clinician do with this information? This chapter will suggest that health professionals are increasingly on solid ground as they attempt to address spiritual issues in patient care. I will describe how this may be done, when it may be done, and what clinicians might expect as a result. The implications are vast, so I will also refer readers to the second edition of *Spirituality in Patient Care* for a far more in-depth discussion.[1]

## WHY DO THIS?

Health professionals are very busy. They might reasonably ask why precious time should be devoted to assessing and addressing patients' spiritual needs. I provide several reasons below.

The first is that many patients are religious, and the majority would like it their faith be considered in their health care. Mrs. Harris lived to be one hundred and one years old and was healthy most of her life. But in her last few years, she had to see more and more doctors, and several times had to be admitted to the hospital. Research shows that many patients like Mrs. Harris—older, female, sicker, and religious—would like to have their religious needs recognized and addressed by their health-care providers.[2] For example, Mrs. Harris might be worried about her diagnosis and want some religious literature to read or someone to pray with. If she didn't get better very soon and was suffering a lot from pain or other physical symptoms, she might start having some religious struggles—wondering why God was allowing her to suffer so, whether she had done anything wrong to deserve this, why God wasn't answering her prayers, why her church friends had stopped calling. She might like to talk with someone about these concerns.

Unless someone asks Mrs. Harris about these kinds of spiritual issues, she might not bring them up, even if they were bothering her a great deal. She might feel too embarrassed to do so with health professionals, since she wouldn't want to offend them or make them feel uncomfortable. As referred to previously, a study of hospitalized patients in Chicago found that 76 percent of medical patients and 88 percent of psychiatric patients had three or more religious needs.[3] Only about one in five hospitalized patients (10 to 30 percent), however, has an opportunity to see a chaplain, and most other health-care professionals are not addressing such needs (fewer than 10 percent of physicians regularly do so).[4] It should not be surprising, then, that failure to meet emotional and spiritual needs is one of the most common complaints of patients on post-hospitalization surveys.[5]

The second reason why health professionals should talk to patients about their spiritual needs is that religion influences patients' ability to cope with illness. As we saw in chapters 4 and 5, up to 90 percent of patients in some areas of the country use religious beliefs to help them to cope when physical illness strikes, and patients who use religion in this way seem truly to cope better than other patients.[6] Because a person's ability to cope may affect motivation toward self-care, willingness to cooperate with planned treatments, and ability to comply with medical therapies, this makes it important for health-care professionals to know something about how the patient is coping. Without such information, it will be difficult to support patients and maximize their coping abilities.

The third reason for addressing spiritual needs is that religious beliefs and practices may influence medical outcomes. Given the adverse effects of stress on the body, when patients' spiritual and emotional needs are unmet, this is likely to affect their immune, endocrine, and cardiovascular systems in ways that could influence the way they respond to surgical and medical treatments (see chapter 3). Such effects on physical outcomes, in addition to the influence of negative emotions on treatment adherence, medication compliance, and motivation toward self-care, are likely to directly or indirectly affect the patient's medical condition (see chapters 4, 8, 9, and 10).

The fourth reason for learning about and addressing spiritual needs is that patients are often isolated from other sources of religious help. People may be hospitalized far away from their faith communities, and long travel distances may prevent clergy and church members from visiting them. Furthermore, clergy may not have the time to visit every patient who is in the hospital and certainly will be limited in the frequency of such visits and the time spent with the patient. Clergy have many other responsibilities besides hospital ministry. Their schedules are usually as packed as those of physicians and nurses. Finally, clergy (and certainly lay church members) may not have the training to address the unique spiritual needs of patients with medical or psychiatric illness. Those needs are quite different from the needs of healthy people. Finally, outside clergy and lay volunteers don't typically work with or know the medical or nursing staff that is caring for patients and certainly won't have access to their medical records. The end result is that patients are often isolated from the kinds of spiritual support that they really need support that is tailored to their specific medical condition.

Fifth, religious beliefs and rituals may conflict with or otherwise influence the medical decisions that patients make, particularly when they are seriously ill. This has been demonstrated in study after study—in patients with cancer, serious lung disease, in end-of-life situations, and in patients from fundamentalist Christian groups, Jehovah witnesses, nonmainstream religious groups, and members of other world religions such as Islam, Buddhism, and Hinduism.[7] Clinicians cannot practice culturally appropriate, whole-person health care without some knowledge of how these beliefs and related rituals influence the care that patients want and will affect their medical decisions during hospitalization and after discharge. Religious beliefs may also influence the threshold at which patients will seek medical or psychiatric care, as exemplified by Christian Scientists, who may shun medical care, or fundamentalist Christians, who may avoid psychiatric care.[8]

Sixth, religious beliefs and commitments influence the type of health care and monitoring that a patient receives in the community after he or she leaves the hospital or doctor's office. Patients in supportive faith communities often have people from those communities call them, visit them, provide emotional support to them, give them rides to the doctor's office, check to be sure they are taking their medicine, ensure that they have adequate meals, and so forth. Health-care professionals need to know if that is the case or, alternatively, if patients will return to a single-room apartment where no one will visit or call on them, express care, or help them out, which may cause them to give up, discontinue their medication, and stop rehabilitation efforts.

Seventh, medical, nursing, and psychiatric training programs are now required to ensure that all graduates provide culturally sensitive health care, which includes care that is sensitive to deeply held religious beliefs. As a result, the Joint Commission for the Accreditation of Hospital Organizations (JCAHO) requires that a spiritual history be taken and documented on every patient admitted to an acute-care hospital or a nursing home or who receives services from home-health agencies. This is a requirement, and the minimal information that must be acquired and documented has been established by JCAHO and is presented on its Web site.[9] That minimal requirement is not met when an admissions clerk or nurse checks a few boxes that indicate whether patients are Catholic,

Protestant, Jewish, or other, and whether or not they want to see a chaplain (the usual procedure in most hospitals today).

Thus, there are many reasons why health-care professionals need to assess and address the spiritual needs of patients and cannot leave this entirely up to chaplains or other clergy. The patient is a unique person with physical, psychological, social, and spiritual needs that must be addressed if health care is to be maximized and the whole person treated.

## How to Do This

How do health professionals go about integrating spirituality into patient care in a sensitive and sensible manner? As a physician, I recognize that time is short and that there are dozens of other areas of patient care that are competing for our time and attention. For the reasons listed above, however, I am asking health professionals to take a brief, screening spiritual history and refer patients with spiritual needs to those who are trained to address them. Health professionals should also be open to discussing issues related to religion or spirituality with patients as the situation warrants (although this should not replace the spiritual history or appropriate referral). Praying with patients is another possibility, if the clinician is open to this and if the patient requests it. Finally, establishing working relationships with the faith community is something that all health professionals can do. I address each of these areas below.

### Taking a Spiritual History

The spiritual history not only collects vital information needed for the care of the patient but also lets the patient know that this is a topic that he or she can talk about with the health professional if the need arises. For a long time, spirituality has been off-limits in the conversations that occur in medical settings. As a result, many health professionals feel uncomfortable discussing such issues, and patients recognize this. Spiritual needs get ignored and swept under the carpet, as if they had no impact or were solely the province of the religious professional.

Physicians, as leaders of the health-care team, should be responsible for taking the screening spiritual history and making the referral. The information learned from the spiritual history has everything to do with the medical care of the patient and the medical decisions that will be made during the course of treatment. This cannot be deferred to a nurse or a chaplain. If, however, the physician does not take a spiritual history, then the responsibility falls to the nurse; if the nurse fails to do so, then it goes to the social worker; if the social worker doesn't do it, then the spiritual history should be done by anyone else involved in the care of the patient.

The screening spiritual history can be quite brief and should take no longer than two or three minutes to complete. This is different from the comprehensive assessment that a chaplain does. I have developed a screening spiritual history for medical patients that consists of the following four questions (called CSI-MEMO, for short):[10]

1. Do your religious/spiritual beliefs provide Comfort, or are they a source of Stress?
2. Do you have spiritual beliefs that might Influence your medical decisions?
3. Are you a MEMber of a religious or spiritual community, and is it supportive to you?
4. Do you have any Other spiritual needs that you'd like someone to address?

The responses to the spiritual history should be documented in a special place in the medical record where everyone on the health-care team can see this information. If patients are referred to professional chaplains for follow-up, then this is where the chaplains would write their notes describing what was done to meet the patient's spiritual needs and any further interventions that might be needed. At this time, it is unclear whether patients should be informed that what they say to health-care chaplains or non chaplain health professionals about spiritual matters may be documented in their medical record. Infroming patients of such documentation is not typically done for other health information acquired by health professionals caring for the patient. Whether information about spiritual matters should be in a different category of protected health information than other health information is debatable.

Before taking the spiritual history, the health professional should carefully explain to the patient the reason that such questions are being asked. Without providing such an explanation beforehand, the patient may misinterpret the intentions of the health professional and begin to panic. In the recent past, the only time a health professional spoke to the patient about religion was when the patient's case was hopeless or far advanced, and nothing else could be done. Therefore, the health professional should explain that the reason for the spiritual history is in order to provide care that is sensitive to patients' cultural and spiritual beliefs and that these questions are required (by JCAHO) for every patient. Patients should be reassured that this has nothing to do with the type or severity of their medical condition, and that it is routine and being doing with everyone.

Because this is a personal and private area for many and because patients will hold a wide assortment of religious beliefs and practices in today's pluralistic health-care settings, it is essential that health professionals *respect, support,* and *value* the beliefs and practices of the patient (especially when those beliefs are different from those of the health professional and even when they seem to be at odds with the medical-treatment plan). This is not a time to try to change patients' religious beliefs (or lack of belief) or to argue with them over religious matters (see below).

The purpose of the spiritual history is to identify spiritual needs that may impact the health care of the patient. Once those needs are identified, the health professional without pastoral training should not feel obligated to address those needs. Instead, the health professional should acknowledge the importance of those spiritual needs and their potential impact on the medical or psychological condition of the patient and then refer that patient to a professional health-care chaplain, who can then assess and address those needs in a competent and comprehensive manner.

## Referring to Chaplains

There is an increasing movement in U.S. hospitals to hire board-certified professional health-care chaplains. Today, about 40 percent of chaplains in the 54–64 percent of hospitals with paid chaplains are board-certified. To be board-certified, a chaplain must have four years of college, three years of divinity school, one to two years of clinical pastoral education (residency in a hospital setting), be recommended by his or her denomination, and then pass a written and an oral board examination. He or she must then obtain fifty hours of continuing education credits every year, ten of which must be approved continuing education by the Association of Professional Chaplains (or another accredited national chaplaincy body). With these credentials and ongoing training to stay updated, chaplains are the true experts at assessing spiritual needs and providing spiritual care in medical settings.

Professional chaplains don't preach to patients about religion or even pray with patients unless requested. Rather, they are trained to walk alongside patients, wherever those patients are in their spiritual journey (which patients are allowed to define, and it may have nothing to do with religion). Chaplains are trained to deal with patients from many different religious backgrounds and those with no religious background. Thus, today's professional chaplain is well trained and prepared to address the spiritual and emotional needs that patients experience when they are sick and in the hospital. For that reason, they should be fully utilized for most spiritual issues that arise during a screening spiritual history.

There is some question about whether consent should be obtained from the patient before referral to a chaplain. Hospitals and health professionals vary on whether or not such consent is obtained. Some patients, however, will be reluctant to see a chaplain. This reluctance usually comes from lack of knowledge about what a chaplain does. Most patients (and most health professionals for that matter) think that a chaplain is simply a minister who prays with patients, talks about religion, performs religious rituals, takes confessions, administers last rites, and conducts chapel services. While the chaplain may do all of these (as the patient directs), he or she does a lot more as well—often simply visiting with patients and talking with them about issues that are important to them. This may involve social, psychological, or spiritual issues, topics that most health professionals these days don't have time for. Therefore, the clinician may need to explain to the patient what a chaplain does and encourage the patient to accept the referral, given the potential impact that unmet spiritual needs may have on the patient's illness and its outcome. Of course, if the patient is not religious, then special care should be taken not to push too hard since coercion must be avoided.

## Praying with Patients

Some health professionals, based on their level of comfort, may be open to praying with patients. No health professional, however, should feel obligated to pray with patients. A brief prayer said by the health professional, however, can be very meaningful to the religious patient and may be one of the most powerful psychosocial interventions that a health professional can do. Although the patient should usually initiate the request for prayer, many patients are not aware that this is even an option and may be scared to ask their health professionals for fear of offending them.

Therefore, I suggest the following. If the health professional has taken a complete spiritual history, if the patient is religious and prayer is important in coping, and if the health professional is willing to pray with the patient, then he or she should let the patient know that he or she is open to praying and encourage the patient, if the patient wants, to bring up the request for prayer at some future visit (not at present, however, to avoid coercion). This way the patient always initiates the request for prayer and forcing prayer on a patient becomes less of an issue. Before praying, the health professional should always ask the patient what she wants to pray for. This should never be assumed and may help to reveal what the patient's most important priority is at this time. The prayer should be short (less than 30 seconds), comforting, and supportive.

### Establish Relationships with Faith Community

All health professionals, whether they are religious or not, should be open to establishing relationships with faith communities and faith-community leaders, who may have a significant influence on the kind of support and care that patients receive in the community. Such relationships may simply involve taking a few minutes to get to know local ministers, priests, rabbis, or imams when they are visiting patients in the hospital. Even better would be participating in a monthly or bimonthly clergy–clinician seminar, which may include a lunch and a guest speaker on a topic of mutual interest. The Pastoral Care Department usually coordinates such meetings. Health professionals can also agree to give a talk at a Sunday school class on a health-related topic. Such relationships often foster the development of referral networks.

## WHEN TO DO THIS

As described above, there are many practical ways that health professionals can address the spiritual needs of patients. In fact, all interactions with patients can be carried out in spiritually sensitive ways, providing treatment in a compassionate, kind, and caring manner that is focused on the individual person and his or her unique needs. This implicit way of providing spiritual care can be done without mentioning a word about spirituality and without taking any extra time specifically to address spiritual issues. Every interaction with the patient can be carried out in this manner. This, of course, cannot replace the time it will take explicitly to address spiritual issues.

So when can busy health professionals explicitly address spiritual issues with patients? For most clinicians, this will involve taking the time to conduct a screening spiritual history. The best time to do this is not during a ten-minute office visit for an acute medical problem. Rather, the spiritual history should be taken when there is more time with the patient and when spiritual issues are relevant. Admission to the acute-care hospital (or a nursing home) is an ideal time. This is when the clinician usually has an opportunity to do a more complete assessment. The social history, which comes after the medical or psychiatric history, is the best time to inquire about spiritual issues. After asking the patient about sources of support (family, friends, etc.), it is quite natural to inquire about religious affiliation, potential conflicts with or influences of religious beliefs on medical care, faith-community involvement, and other relevant questions as described above (CSI-MEMO). Not all of this information needs to be collected at one time if the clinician is rushed. Sometimes a single question will be enough in the short term, such as, "Do you have any spiritual needs or concerns related to your health?" This will elicit any urgent spiritual needs that can then be addressed or referred on to pastoral care.

A spiritual history can also be taken during a well-patient examination or yearly physical. There is usually more time set aside for such visits, and these interactions often focus on disease prevention and health promotion. This may also be an opportunity when the clinician asks about the family, other support systems, coping with stress at work, or other health problems. A few questions about spiritual needs, in the context of asking about other sources of support, may be naturally included here. Another time for addressing spiritual issues is when a stressful diagnosis or serious prognosis is being discussed, as in a patient with a terminal or chronic illness. Discussions related to end-of-life issues should always include a spiritual history. However, the spiritual history should not be reserved only for end-of-life discussions, but for all patients with serious, chronic, or disabling diseases or conditions that may challenge their ability to cope.

## WHAT RESULTS FROM THIS?

What might result from assessing and addressing the spiritual needs of patients? How will patients react? Will they be offended or upset? Besides the benefits of uncovering beliefs that may conflict with medical care or influence medical decisions, what direct effect might addressing the patient's spirituality have on his or her health outcome? Although there is not a lot of systematic research on the consequences of taking a spiritual history or praying with patients, there are many anecdotal reports and at least one randomized clinical trial.

Religious patients often deeply appreciate it when their healthcare provider inquires about, acknowledges the value of, and supports their religious beliefs and when that provider makes an effort to consider and integrate those beliefs as part of health care. The nonreligious patient or the patient with conflicts in the religious area will likely want to avoid such discussions, and some degree of resistance may be encountered. That resistance, however, is not usually very strong unless health professionals persist in pursuing this topic even after the patient has made it clear that doing so makes him or her feel uncomfortable (see below).

There has been at least one randomized clinical trial that provides information to help guide clinicians in this area. Kristeller and colleagues conducted a clinical trial to assess the effect of a physician-administered spiritual history intervention in 118 consecutive oncology outpatients.[11] Physicians involved in the study were four oncologists: two were Christians, one was Hindu, and one was a Sikh. Over 80 percent of patients were Christian, and 15 percent indicated no religious affiliation. Patients were alternately assigned to either the intervention group or a usual care control group. Alternate, rather than random, assignment was done in order to minimize the burden on any one oncologist. The investigators, who used the OASIS questionnaire, acknowledged that the intervention was more than just taking a spiritual history:

> The OASIS model uses a brief semi-structured standardized format that utilizes open-ended questions based on principles of patient-centered counseling and relationship-centered care. Such an approach communicates the physician's interest in the patient's experience, and also encourages individuals to consider these issues more deeply themselves. It is important to distinguish the conceptual framework of this approach from that of taking a medical or spiritual "history," in which the goal is to collect information about the patient for the purpose of providing future care. Rather, the structure is intended to facilitate communication between the patient and physician and to empower the patient, if need be, to more fully consider his or her own issues and resources in this domain.[12]

This intervention took an average of six minutes to administer and increased the length of the outpatient visit from 13.1 minutes to 14.8 minutes. Results revealed that, in most cases (85 percent), physicians were comfortable administering the intervention and the majority of patients (76 percent) thought it was useful. Standard scales measuring quality of life, depression, and patient–physician communication were administered at baseline and then repeated three weeks after the intervention. On the three-week follow-up evaluation, results indicated that patients who received the intervention had a greater reduction in depressive symptoms, compared to the control group. In addition, patients receiving the intervention had a greater sense of interpersonal caring from the physician and an increase in their functional well-being, compared to control patients.

In many respects, this study maximized the potential for conflict when taking a spiritual history. First, a significant proportion of patients (15 percent) had no religious affiliation and likely represented a group who did not perceive these issues to be very important to them. Second, half of the oncologists delivering the intervention were from religious backgrounds different from those of the patients. Finally, the intervention was more extensive and aggressive than simply taking a spiritual history, as the investigators acknowledge above. Despite this potential for conflict, however, few difficulties were encountered. Most patients and physicians were comfortable with the process, and the results were clearly positive in terms of the measured outcomes.

## WHAT NOT TO DO

There is much that health professionals can do in terms of taking a spiritual history, supporting patients' beliefs, referring spiritual needs to professional chaplains, perhaps saying a short prayer if requested by the patient, and developing relationships with local chaplains and clergy. However, there are also boundaries that health professionals should not cross. I will identify five clear "do nots" in this area.

First, health professionals should not prescribe religion to nonreligious patients or actively proselytize. This involves coercion and possibly represents an ethical and human rights violation.

Second, and similarly, health professionals should not continue a spiritual history if the patient is not religious and indicates discomfort or resistance to such questioning. All interventions in this area, including the spiritual history, must be "patient-centered" and guided by patient choice.

Third, clinicians should not pray with a patient before taking an in-depth spiritual history and unless the patient asks. Patients from certain religious denominations may be offended by a health professional offering to pray if that person is not from their own religious background. Also, patients may not be able to refuse a clinician's request to pray because of the authority status of the health professional. Patients often want to please doctors or nurses and may not want to offend them since they are making health-care decisions.

Fourth, health professionals without religious training should usually not provide spiritual counsel or advice to patients. Spiritual needs can be very complex and may be intertwined with psychological issues and social conflicts. Addressing spiritual needs requires training on how to do so sensitively and effectively. Just as physicians, nurses, and social workers require special training to do what they do, the same is true for those professionals who provide spiritual care. After obtaining consent, the clinician should refer patients with spiritual needs to professional chaplains or pastoral counselors.

Finally, health professionals should never argue with patients about religious beliefs, even when those beliefs conflict with medical or nursing care. It is always better to learn about the patient's religious beliefs and seek understanding on how those beliefs could affect patients' medical decisions. Whenever possible, the health-care environment should be altered to accommodate religious rituals and other practices. Arguments about beliefs almost always upset patients and family members and lead to alienation and noncompliance. If patients sense that health professionals do not respect and value their beliefs, beliefs that give life meaning and provide psychological and social support, then they will view the health professional as an adversary, which will interfere with future interactions. Alternatively, if the clinician shows respect and honor for the patient's beliefs, then it is much more likely that the patient will eventually come around to the clinician's way of thinking and become more receptive to recommended treatment.

## CONCLUSIONS

Research showing that religious beliefs influence coping with illness, affect medical decisions, and likely influence medical outcomes is beginning to accumulate. This makes it more and more difficult to ignore the spiritual needs of patients. Sensible clinical applications now exist that have the potential to improve overall patient care, enhance patient satisfaction, and benefit medical and psychological outcomes. Health professionals should take a spiritual history on all patients with chronic, disabling, or serious illness and document this in the medical record, referring those with spiritual needs to professional chaplains. Supporting the patient's own religious beliefs, creating a medical environment that allows for important religious rituals, praying with a patient if requested, and welcoming interactions with the faith community are other ways that health professionals can integrate spirituality into patient care. Clinical applications must always be patient-centered and guided by patient choice, and there are important boundaries that health professionals should not cross.

## CHAPTER 12
## Final Thoughts

THERE IS MUCH DISCUSSION today about the role of spirituality in medicine. The research that is coming out in peer-reviewed medical, public health, sociology, psychology, nursing, social work, and rehabilitation science journals suggests that there are relationships between religious involvement and both mental and physical health. Much more research is needed to understand how these relationships operate and whether they are causal (i.e., that religious involvement actually causes better health). There is mounting evidence from randomized clinical trials and prospective studies that religious beliefs and practices have positive effects on coping and on speeding remission from emotional disorders, such as anxiety and depression. By improving coping, giving hope, and fostering a sense of meaning and purpose during difficult life circumstances, religious beliefs have the potential to impact not only mental health but physical health as well, given what we know about the impact of negative emotions and stress on physiological systems (immune, endocrine, and cardiovascular), disease outcomes, and longevity.

Even if religious involvement were completely unrelated to physical health and medical outcomes, however, integrating spirituality into patient care should still be a priority. Because so many medical patients have spiritual needs, spiritual conflicts, or derive comfort from religious beliefs and traditions, this makes a strong argument for training health professionals to assess, respect, and make accommodations for patients' spiritual beliefs and practices. It also emphasizes the importance of having strong Pastoral Care Departments in hospitals to ensure that someone meets the spiritual needs of patients in a way that is sensitive and culturally appropriate.

Thus, both a solid research base and common sense argue that the religious and spiritual beliefs of patients are linked in one way or another to their health and well-being. Learning to respect the power of those beliefs and utilize them to speed the patient's healing and recovery of wholeness, then, should be a priority for modern medicine and health care.

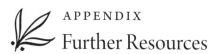

# APPENDIX
## Further Resources

## Key Research Studies
### (in order of publication year)

### Mental Health

**Moberg, D. O. "Religious activities and personal adjustment in old age."**
*Journal of Social Psychology*, 43 (1956): 261–67.
One of the first systematic research studies on the religion–mental health relationship. This study involved a survey of 219 persons over age 65 who resided in seven institutions (five old-age homes) in the Minneapolis–St. Paul area. Assessed religiosity and personal adjustment. Religiosity measured by 11 items (church membership, present attendance, present attendance compared to age-55 attendance, age-12 attendance, positions or church offices held, listening to religious radio, reading the Bible, reading other religious books, private prayer, saying grace at meals, frequency of family prayers). Religiosity was positively related to adjustment ($r = 0.59$, SE .04, highly significant); those with high religious scores ($n = 86$) were compared to those with low religious scores ($n = 41$), again showing greater personal adjustment in the former. Nineteen high and nineteen low religiosity subjects were matched on multiple indices and compared, with high religiosity subjects showing greater adjustment.

**Blazer, D. G., and E. Palmore. "Religion and Aging in a Longitudinal Panel."** *The Gerontologist* 16 (1976): 82–85.
One of the first cohort studies using a well-known sample (Duke Longitudinal Study I) and state-of-the-art methods and analyses (for the mid-1970s). The religion subscale of Chicago Inventory of Activities and Attitudes was used to measure religious activity (church attendance, listening to religious radio/TV, reading Bible/devotional books); religious attitudes were based on agreement or disagreement with statements indicative of religion's impor-

tance or extent of comfort derived from religion. Over 20 years, religious activity gradually decreased over time, although religious attitudes remained stable. Neither religious activities nor religious attitudes were related to mortality. However, religious activities were significantly related to happiness (especially in men and persons over 70), feeling useful (especially for those in manual occupations and over age 70), and personal adjustment (especially in those with manual occupations and in males). Religious attitudes were unrelated to happiness but were related to usefulness (especially those in manual occupations). Correlations increased during the later rounds of the study, suggesting increasing importance of religion for well-being over time.

**Koenig, H. G., J. N. Kvale, and C. Ferrel. "Religion and Well-being in Later Life." *The Gerontologist* 28 (1988): 18–28.**
One of the largest and most detailed studies on religious characteristics and well-being to date. This was a cross-sectional survey of 836 persons ages 55 or older in the midwestern United States., consisting of senior-center participants, church and synagogue members, retired nuns, and geriatric medical outpatients. Multiple-item measures of organizational religiosity (ORA), nonorganizational religiosity (NORA), and intrinsic religiosity (IR) were used. The seventeen-item Philadelphia Center Morale Scale was used to assess well-being. ORA, NORA, and IR were all significantly and positively related to well-being at correlations ranging from 0.16–0.26. After controlling for the effects of health, social support, and financial status, relationships with well-being remained significant (p < 0.0001). Effects were greatest in women (17 percent of explained variance in well-being) and in persons aged 75 or older (25 percent of the explained variance).

**Propst, L. R., R. Ostrom, P. Watkins, et al. "Comparative Efficacy of Religious and Nonreligious Cognitive-Behavior Therapy for the Treatment of Clinical Depression in Religious Individuals." *Journal of Consulting and Clinical Psychology* 60 (1992): 94–103.**
First large-scale randomized clinical trial examining effectiveness of using religion-based cognitive-behavioral psychotherapy (RCT) versus traditional CBT (NRCT) versus ordinary pastoral counseling (PCT) versus wait-list control (WLC) in the treatment of fifty-nine depressed religious patients. RCT was used employing Christian religious rationales, religious arguments to counter irrational thoughts, and religious imagery. RCT resulted in significantly lower post-treatment depression scores than WLC for Beck Depression Inventory (BDI). RCT and PCT showed trends toward lower post-treatment Hamilton Depression Rating Scale (HRSD) scores than WLC. Finally,

RCT group demonstrated significantly better social adjustment scores (SAS) than did WLC (p < 0.001). RCT patients receiving therapy from nonreligious therapists reported significantly lower post-treatment BDI scores than both WLC group (p < 0.001) and NRCT group with nonreligious therapists (p < 0.02); similar findings present for HRDS and SAS scores.

**Koenig, H. G., H. J. Cohen, D. G. Blazer, et al. "Religious Coping and Depression in Elderly Hospitalized Medically Ill Men."** *American Journal of Psychiatry* **149 (1992): 1693–1700.**
One of the first studies of religion and depression published in a major psychiatric journal. See chapter 5 for details.

**Levin, J. S., L. M. Chatters, and R. J. Taylor. "Religious Effects on Health Status and Life Satisfaction among Black Americans."** *Journals of Gerontology Series B: Psychological Sciences and Social Sciences* **50B (1995): S154–S163.**
One of the first studies to show an association between life satisfaction and religious activity using the new statistical method, structural equation modeling. Investigators used data from a national probability sample of 1,848 black Americans (National Survey of Black Americans). They split the sample into two equal groups for analysis. Multi-item measures of public, private, and subjective religiosity were used. Using Linear Standard Relations (LISREL), found public religious activity was associated with physical health and life satisfaction after controlling for age, gender, education, marital status, employment status, geographical region, and urban-versus-rural residence. After controlling for initial health status, public religiosity remained significantly associated with life satisfaction in both of the split samples. Subjective religiosity was also significantly related to life satisfaction in both subsamples in uncontrolled analysis. These associations were present in all age groups (under age 30, ages 30–55, and over age 55 years).

**Kennedy, G. J., H. R. Kelman, C. Thomas, et al. "The Relation of Religious Preference and Practice to Depressive Symptoms among 1,855 Older Adults."** *Journals of Gerontology Series B: Psychological Sciences and Social Sciences* **51B (1996): P301–P308.**
One of the largest prospective cohort studies involving large numbers of Jews and Catholics from New York City. Studied a random sample of 1,855 older community residents (40 percent Jewish and 47 percent Catholic) in the north Bronx. Jews were more likely to have had a mental health visit than Catholics or other faiths, more likely to use psychotropic medication, more likely to score high on depressive symptoms. Using logistic regression,

investigators reported that Jews were 75 percent more likely than persons of other religious affiliations to have depression (p < 0.0001). Frequent religious attendance was associated with lower rates of depression in Catholics, but not Jews; Catholics who attended services once a month or more were over 60 percent less likely to be depressed (p < 0.0001). When followed over twenty-four months, Jews were more likely to experience an emergence of depression than Catholics or other faiths, a difference that persisted after controlling for six other predictors of depression in a multivariate model, and to have persistent depression if they were depressed at the start of the study.

**Koenig, H. G., L. K. George, and B. L. Peterson. "Religiosity and Remission from Depression in Medically Ill Older Patients."** *American Journal of Psychiatry* **155 (1998): 536–42.**
The first study to show that religiosity was related to recovery from a depressive disorder, diagnosed using a structured psychiatric interview. See chapter 5 for details.

**Braam, A. W., P. Van Den Eeden, M. J. Prince, et al. "Religion as a Cross-cultural Determinant of Depression in Elderly Europeans: Results from the EURODEP Collaboration."** *Psychological Medicine* **31, no. 5 (2001): 803–14.**
One of the largest studies in Europe showing a relationship between religion and depression. First, investigators studied associations between church attendance, religious denomination, and depression in six EURODEP study centers located in five countries involving 8,398 persons. Second, the relationship between "religious climate" and depressive symptoms was determined based on data from the European Values Survey administered to 17,739 persons from 11 European countries. Investigators found a lower prevalence of depressive symptoms in regular church attendees, an effect that was most evident among Catholics. In addition, fewer depressive symptoms were found among older women in countries with high rates of regular church attendance (generally, Catholic countries). Levels of depressive symptoms were significantly higher among older men in Protestant countries. Researchers concluded that religious practices were associated with less depression in elderly Europeans.

**Fontana, A., and R. Rosenheck. "Trauma, Change in Strength of Religious Faith, and Mental Health Service Use among Veterans Treated for PTSD."** *Journal of Nervous and Mental Disease* **192 (2004): 579–84.**
First large study to show consequences of not addressing spiritual injury in patients with Post-Traumatic Stress Disorder (PTSD). Examining 1,385

veterans from the Vietnam War (95 percent), World War II, and/or the Korean conflict involved in outpatient or inpatient PTSD programs, investigators from the VA National Center for PTSD and Yale University School of Medicine examined relationships between veterans' exposure to traumatic stress, PTSD, changes in religious faith, and use of mental health services. Structural equation modeling used to show that a weakened religious faith as a result of traumatic war experiences independently predicted great use of VA mental health services—independent of severity of PTSD symptoms and level of social functioning. Weakening of religious faith (spiritual injury) was one of the strongest predictor of veterans' seeking mental health services over the years, even stronger than the severity of the clinical symptoms themselves.

**Koenig, H. G. "Religion and Depression in Older Medical Inpatients."** *American Journal of Geriatric Psychiatry* **15, no. 4 (2007): 282–91.**
Largest study to date among medical inpatients of the relationship between depression and religious involvement. One thousand medical inpatients over age 50 at Duke University Medical Center (DUMC) and three community hospitals were identified with depressive disorder using a structured psychiatric interview. Religious characteristics of these depressed patients were then compared to those of 428 nondepressed patients in a concurrent study at DUMC, controlling for demographic, health, and social factors. Relationships to severity and type of depression were also examined among depressed patients themselves. Depressed patients were more likely to indicate no religious affiliation, less likely to affiliate with fundamentalist denominations, more likely to describe themselves as "spiritual but not religious," less likely to pray or read scripture, and scored lower on intrinsic religiosity. Among depressed patients, lower religious attendance, less prayer, less scripture reading, and lower intrinsic religiosity were associated with more symptoms.

**Koenig, H. G. "Religion and Remission of Depression in Medical Inpatients with Heart Failure/Pulmonary Disease."** *Journal of Nervous and Mental Disease* **195, no. 5 (2007):389–95**
Largest prospective study to date of the impact of religious involvement on remission of depression in medical inpatients. See chapter 5 for details.

### Physical Health

**Comstock, G. W., and K. B. Partridge. "Church Attendance and Health."** *Journal of Chronic Disease* **25 (1972): 665–72.**
One of the first studies to find an association between religious activity and health. Investigators compared death rates for a three-to-six-year period for

24,245 frequent church attendees and 30,603 infrequent attendees who participated in the Washington County, Maryland, 1963 census. Reported a higher relative risk of dying for infrequent versus frequent attendees. Infrequent attendees had an increased relative risk (RR) of 2.1 for death from atherosclerotic heart disease in women aged 45–64 years; RR = 2.3 for death from pulmonary emphysema (both genders); RR = 3.9 for death from cirrhosis of the liver; and RR = 2.1 for death from suicide. Adjustments for age, sex, and race did not make major differences in relative risks. Investigators noted that these associations may be due to the fact that ill people cannot attend church frequently and that diminution of the effect over time would be consistent with this kind of spurious effect. The broad range of effects prompted the authors to conclude that the relationship of church attendance to health is nonspecific rather than causal.

**Goldbourt, U., S. Yaari, and J. H. Medalie. "Factors Predictive of Long-term Coronary Heart Disease Mortality among 10,059 Male Israeli Civil Servants and Municipal Employees."** *Cardiology* 82 (1993): 100–21.
Largest, longest follow-up study of religiousness and death rates from coronary artery disease (CAD), a twenty-three-year prospective cohort study of 10,059 Jewish immigrant males aged 40 or over working as civil servants or municipal employees in Israel. Religiousness, measured by three items (religious versus secular education; self-definition as orthodox, traditional, or secular; and frequency of synagogue attendance), was used to create an index. Most religious group (20 percent) had lowest rate of mortality from coronary artery disease (CAD) (38 versus 61 per 10,000) and other causes (135 versus 168 per 10,000) than did nonbelievers. The risk of death from CAD among the most religious group was 20 percent less than others; results remained significant after controlling for age, systolic blood pressure, cholesterol, smoking, diabetes, body mass index, and baseline CAD.

**Oxman, T. E., D. H. Freeman, and E. D. Manheimer. "Lack of Social Participation or Religious Strength and Comfort as Risk Factors for Death after Cardiac Surgery in the Elderly."** *Psychosomatic Medicine* 57 (1995): 5–15.
The first prospective study to examine effects of religious involvement on death rates following open-heart surgery. Investigators followed 232 patients age 55 or over at Dartmouth Medical Center following elective cardiac surgery. Subjects were assessed one and six months after surgery; religious variables included affiliation, religious attendance, strength and comfort from religion, number of people known in congregation, and self-rated religiousness.

Logistical regression determined five major predictors of mortality during the six months after surgery: previous cardiac surgery, severity of impairments in physical functioning, age over 70, participation in social groups, and strength or comfort from religion. After adjusting for other predictors, those with lack of strength or comfort from religion were more than three times more likely to die (OR 3.25, 95 percent CI 1.09-9.72). Among the 72 who had both high social group participation and high religious strength and comfort, only 2.5 percent died, compared with over 21 percent of the 49 subjects with no group participation or deriving no strength and comfort from religion.

**Kark, J. D., G. Shemi, Y. Friedlander, O. Martin, O. Manor, and S. H. Blondheim. "Does Religious Observance Promote Health? Mortality in Secular versus Religious Kibbutzim in Israel."** *American Journal of Public Health* 86 (1996): 341–46.

The importance of this study is that it completely controlled for the effects of social factors on association between religion and mortality. This was a sixteen-year historical cohort study of 3,900 persons that compared mortality rates among members of 11 religious kibbutzim with those of members of 11 secular kibbutzim. Careful matching was performed to ensure that secular and religious kibbutzim were as similar as possible in characteristics that might affect mortality. Persons in secular kibbutzim had a mortality risk that was 93 percent greater than members of religious kibbutzim (RH = 1.93, 95 percent CI 1.44-2.59, $p < 0.0001$). This helps to address the criticisms of those who feel the health effects of religion are all due to social support and nothing else. Religious men lived just as long as secular women (i.e., eliminated the gender advantage in survival).

**Strawbridge, W. J., R. D. Cohen, S. J. Shema, and G. A. Kaplan. "Frequent Attendance at Religious Services and Mortality over 28 Years."** *American Journal of Public Health* 87 (1997): 957–61.

This best-designed study of the effects of religious attendance on survival to date. For details, see chapter 9.

**Idler, E. L., and S. V. Kasl. "Religion among Disabled and Nondisabled Elderly Persons, II: Attendance at Religious Services as a Predictor of the Course of Disability."** *Journals of Gerontology Series B: Psychological Sciences and Social Sciences* 52B (1997): S306–S316.

One of the first and best-designed studies of the effects of religious activity on forestalling the development of functional disability in later life.

Koenig, H. G., H. J. Cohen, L. K. George, J. C. Hays, D. B. Larson, and D. G. Blazer. "Attendance at Religious Services, Interleukin-6, and Other Biological Indicators of Immune Function in Older Adults." *International Journal of Psychiatry in Medicine* 27 (1997): 233–50.
First study to report associations between religious activity and biological indicators of immune function/inflammation. For details, see chapter 6.

Koenig, H. G., and D. B. Larson. "Use of Hospital Services, Church Attendance, and Religious Affiliation." *Southern Medical Journal* 91 (1998): 925–32.
One of first studies to show an association between religious involvement and use of inpatient hospital services. Investigators found an inverse relationship between frequency of religious service attendance and likelihood of hospital admission in a sample of 455 older patients. Those who attended church weekly or more often were significantly less likely in the previous year to have been admitted to the hospital, had fewer hospital admissions, and spent fewer days in the hospital than those attending less often; these associations retained their significance after controlling for covariates. Patients unaffiliated with a religious community had significantly longer index hospital stays than those affiliated. Unaffiliated patients spent an average of 25 days in the hospital, compared with 11 days for affiliated patients (p < 0.0001); this association strengthened when physical health and other covariates were controlled.

Hummer, R. A., R. G. Rogers, C. B. Nam, and C. G. Ellison. "Religious Involvement and U.S. Adult Mortality." *Demography* 36 (1999): 273–85.
The largest study of the effects of religious attendance on survival, as of early 2007. For details, see chapter 9.

Helm, H. M., J. C. Hays, E. P. Flint, H. G. Koenig, and D. G. Blazer. "Does Private Religious Activity Prolong Survival? A Six-Year Follow-Up Study of 3,851 Older Adults." *Journals of Gerontology Series A: Biological Sciences and Medical Sciences* 55 (2000): M400–5.
One of few prospective studies showing an effect of prayer on mortality by examining this effect in healthy elders. For details, see chapter 9.

Pargament, K. I., H. G. Koenig, N. Tarakeshwar, and J. Hahn. "Religious Struggle as a Predictor of Mortality among Medically Ill Elderly Patients: A Two-Year Longitudinal Study." *Archives of Internal Medicine* 161 (2001): 1881–85.
First study to show prospectively the negative effects of religious struggle on mortality in medical inpatients. For details, see chapter 9.

Steffen, P. R., and A. L. Hinderliter. "Religious Coping, Ethnicity, and Ambulatory Blood Pressure." *Psychosomatic Medicine* 63, no. 4 (2001): 523–30.
One of first studies to examine effects of religious coping on ambulatory blood pressure. For details, see chapter 7.

Ironson, G., G. F. Solomon, E. G. Balbin, et al. "Spirituality and Religiousness Are Associated with Long Survival, Health Behaviors, Less Distress, and Lower Cortisol in People Living with HIV/AIDS: The IWORSHIP Scale, Its Validity and Reliability." *Annals of Behavioral Medicine* 24 (2002): 34–48.
First study to show that long-term survivors with HIV/AIDS were more religious and to suggest a mechanism (cortisol). For details, see chapter 6.

Lutgendorf, S. K., D. Russell, P. Ullrich, T. B. Harris, and R. Wallace. "Religious Participation, Interleukin-6, and Mortality in Older Adults." *Health Psychology* 23, no. 5 (2004): 465–75.
Replicated the associations between religious activity and immune function (interleukin-6) found in the Duke University study (Koenig et al., 1997) above. Furthermore, linked this association with mortality rate. For details, see chapter 6.

Masters, K. S., R. D. Hill, J. C. Kircher, T. L. Benson, and J. A. Fallon. "Religious Orientation, Aging, and Blood Pressure Reactivity to Interpersonal and Cognitive Stressors." *Annals of Behavioral Medicine* 28, no. 3 (2004):171–78.
One of the best studies examining effects of religious involvement on cardiovascular reactivity. For details, see chapter 7.

Ironson, G., R. Stuetzie, and M. A. Fletcher. "An Increase in Religiousness/Spirituality Occurs after HIV Diagnosis and Predicts Slower Disease Progression over 4 Years in People with HIV." *Journal of General Internal Medicine* 21 (2006): S62–S68.
First study to show prospectively an effect of turning to religion/spirituality on immune function (CD-4 lymphocyte counts) and viral load in HIV-positive patients. For details, see chapter 6.

Hill, T. D., A. M. Burdette, J. L. Angel, and R. J. Angel. "Religious Attendance and Cognitive Functioning among Older Mexican Americans." *Journals of Gerontology Series B: Psychological Sciences and Social Sciences* 61, no. 1 (2006): P3–P9.
One of the best of several studies showing an association between religious activity and slower worsening of cognitive functioning with aging. For details, see chapter 8.

Tully, J., R. M. Viner, P. G. Coen, et al. "Risk and Protective Factors for Meningococcal Disease in Adolescents: Matched Cohort Study." *British Medical Journal* 332, no. 7539 (2006): 445–50.

Researchers prospectively examined the ability of social and biological factors to predict the development of meningococcal disease in adolescents aged fifteen to nineteen years. Cases with meningococcal disease were matched with controls on age and gender. A total of 144 case-control pairs participated in the study (median age 17.6). Among cases, 79 percent were confirmed from microbiological cultures/serology from nose and mouth swabs. Based on multivariate logistic regression modeling, predictors of increased likelihood of meningococcal disease were prior illness, intimate kissing with multiple partners, status as a university student, and preterm birth status. Meningococcal vaccination was inversely associated with disease (OR 0.12, 95 percent CI 0.04-0.37, p < 0.001), as was religious attendance (OR = 0.10, 95 percent CI 0.02-0.58, p = 0.01). Thus, religious attendance was associated with a 90 percent reduced likelihood of having menningococcal disease, equivalent to that of meningococcal vaccination.

## Applications to Clinical Practice

Silvestri, G. A., S. Knittig, et al. "Importance of Faith on Medical Decisions regarding Cancer Care." *Journal of Clinical Oncology* 21 (2003): 1379–82.

Study demonstrates large gap between how patients value and use religion in decision making and how health professionals feel about this. Investigators surveyed one hundred patients with advanced lung cancer, their caregivers, and 257 medical oncologists attending an annual meeting of the American Society of Clinical Oncology. Researchers asked participants to rank the importance of seven factors that might influence treatment decisions on whether to accept chemotherapy. Although patients and family members both ranked "faith in God" as no. 2 (outranked only by the recommendation of the oncologist), oncologists ranked faith in God last (seventh) (p < 0.0001).

Kristeller, J. L., M. Rhodes, L. D. Cripe, and V. Sheets. "Oncologist Assisted Spiritual Intervention Study (OASIS): Patient Acceptability and Initial Evidence of Effects." *International Journal of Psychiatry in Medicine* 35 (2005): 329–47.

First RCT showing an effect of taking a spiritual history on clinical outcomes and patient acceptability. This RCT involved examining the effect of a physician-administered spiritual history intervention in 118 consecutive outpatients with cancer. Physicians involved in the study were four oncologists (two Christian, one Hindu, and one Sikh). Intervention was called the OASIS spiritual history (SH). Results indicated that in most cases (85 percent), physicians were comfortable administering the intervention and the majority of patients (76 percent) thought it was useful. Three weeks after the visit, patients receiving the SH intervention had a significantly greater reduction in depressive symptoms ($p < 0.01$), a greater sense of interpersonal caring from physician ($p < 0.05$), and increased functional well-being ($p < 0.001$), compared with control patients.

Balboni, T. A., L. C. Vanderwerker, S. D. Block, et al. "Religiousness and Spiritual Support among Advanced Cancer Patients and Associations with End-of-Life Treatment Preferences and Quality of Life." *Journal of Clinical Oncology* 25 (2007): 555–60.
One of the best studies showing patients' preferences regarding spiritual care and impact of addressing those preferences. Surveyed 230 patients with advanced cancer and their caregivers in Boston (Coping with Cancer Study at Harvard). Patients rated to what extent either their religious community or the medical system supported their spiritual needs on a scale from 1 (not at all) to 5 (completely supported). Findings indicated that 88 percent of patients said that religion was at least somewhat important. However, just under half (47 percent) said that their spiritual needs were minimally or not at all met by their religious community; furthermore, nearly three-quarters (72 percent) said that their spiritual needs were minimally or not at all met by the medical system (i.e., doctors, nurses, or chaplains). Patients who indicated that either the religious community or the medical system was providing spiritual support reported significantly higher quality of life ($p < 0.0005$). Of nine variables, degree of spiritual support was the second most powerful predictor of quality of life (especially African Americans and Hispanics).

## RESEARCH REVIEW ARTICLES
## (IN ORDER OF PUBLICATION YEAR)

Sanua, V. D. "Religion, Mental Health, and Personality: A Review of Empirical Studies." *American Journal of Psychiatry* 125 (1969): 1203–13.
In this first modern-day review of the research on mental health, the following quote summarizes this reviewer's conclusions: "The contention that religion as an institution has been instrumental in fostering general well-being,

creativity, honesty, liberalism, and other qualities is not supported by empirical data. Both Scott and Godin point out that there are no scientific studies which show that religion is capable of serving mental health" (1203).

**Levin, J. S., and P. L. Schiller. "Is There a Religious Factor in Health?"** *Journal of Religion and Health* 26 (1987): 9–36.
The first comprehensive review article on research examining religion and physical health; reviews studies conducted in the early part of the twentieth century and forward.

**Koenig, H. G. "Research on Religion and Mental Health in Later Life: A Review and Commentary."** *Journal of Geriatric Psychiatry* 23 (1990): 23–53.
The article is one of the first reviews of research on religion and mental health in older adults in a specialty psychiatric journal.

**Larson, D. B., K. A. Sherrill, J. S. Lyons, et al. "Associations between Dimensions of Religious Commitment and Mental Health Reported in the** *American Journal of Psychiatry* **and** *Archives of General Psychiatry:* **1978–1989."** *American Journal of Psychiatry* 149, no. 4 (1992): 557–59.
The article is the first research review (since the Sanua article above) on religion and mental health in a top psychiatric journal.

**Levin, J. S. "Religion and Health: Is There an Association, Is It Valid, and Is It Causal?"** *Social Sciences and Medicine* 38 (1994):1475–82.
Reviews the research and evaluates the quality and meaning of associations reported between religion and physical health.

**Sloan, R. P., E. Bagiella, and T. Powell. "Religion, Spirituality, and Medicine."** *Lancet* 353, no. 9153 (1999): 664–67.
This selective review strongly criticizes the research on religion and physical health.

**McCullough, M. E., W. T. Hoyt, D. B. Larson, H. G. Koenig, and C. Thoresen. "Religious Involvement and Mortality: A Meta-Analytic Review."** *Health Psychology* 19 (2000): 211–22.
The article is the first formal meta-analysis of research on religious involvement and mortality. For details, see chapter 9.

Koenig, H. G. "Religion and Medicine, I–IV." *International Journal of Psychiatry in Medicine* 30 (2000): 385–98; 31 (2001): 97–109; 31 (2001): 217–35; and 31 (2001): 337–52.
This series of four articles summarizes research reported in the *Handbook of Religion and Health* (see below).

Mueller, P. S., D. J. Plevak, and T. A. Rummans. "Religious Involvement, Spirituality, and Medicine: Implications for Clinical Practice." *Mayo Clinic Proceedings* 76 (2001): 1225–35.
Mayo Clinic researchers comprehensively review of the research on religion, spirituality, and health, and its clinical implications.

George, L. K., C. G. Ellison, and D. B. Larson. "Explaining the Relationships between Religious Involvement and Health." *Psychological Inquiry* 13 (2002): 190–200.
Important review article that attempts to explain why religious involvement is related to health. Provides important theory.

Koenig, H. G. "An 83-Year-Old Woman with Chronic Illness and Strong Religious Beliefs." *Journal of the American Medical Association* 288 (2002): 487–93.
This article provides a case report, research review, and discussion of clinical implications as part of the Clinical Crossroads section of *JAMA*.

Powell, L. H., L. Shahabi, and C. E. Thoresen. "Religion and Spirituality: Linkages to Physical Health," *American Psychologist* 58, no. 1 (2003): 36–52.
This article reviews the research on religion and health, taking a conservative and minimalist approach to the research data on physical health.

Koenig, H. G. "Annotated Bibliography of Religion, Spirituality and Medicine." *Southern Medical Journal* 99 (2006): 1189–96.
This article provides an annotated bibliography of recent research on religion, spirituality, and health.

Rew, L., and Y. J. Wong. "A Systematic Review of Associations among Religiosity/Spirituality and Adolescent Health Attitudes and Behaviors." *Journal of Adolescent Health* 38, no. 4 (2006): 433–42.
This review of research on the relationship between religion/spirituality and adolescent attitudes and behaviors is one of the most recent comprehensive treatments of this topic in young persons.

## BOOKS
### (IN ORDER OF PUBLICATION YEAR)

**Koenig, H. G., M. Smiley, and J. Gonzales. *Religion, Health, and Aging.* Westport, CT: Greenwood Press, 1988.**
Provides a comprehensive review and discussion of research and writings on the relationship between religion and health in later life, covering both physical and mental health; numerous cases of older adults using religion to cope are presented, along with original data on relationships between religion, aging and health, much of which has not been published elsewhere (includes measurement tools).

**Koenig, H. G. *Aging and God: Spiritual Paths to Mental Health in Midlife and Later Years.* New York: Haworth Press, 1994.**
This book, over 500 pages, provides an in-depth treatment of religion and mental health in older adults, updating research since the 1988 book was published (focusing now on older medical inpatients). Sections on history, research, case reports, and clinical applications are presented.

**Levin, J. S., ed. *Religion in Aging and Health.* Thousand Oaks, CA: Sage Publications, 1994.**
Preeminent researcher and skilled writer, Dr. Levin serves as editor for this book with chapters by experts in the scholarly field of religion and aging.

**Shafranske, E. P., ed. *Religion and the Clinical Practice of Psychology.* Washington, DC: American Psychological Association, 1996.**
This massive textbook for psychologists addresses every aspect of addressing religious issues in clinical practice.

**Pargament, K. I. *The Psychology of Religion and Coping.* New York: Guilford Press, 1997.**
As the world expert on religious coping, Dr. Pargament reviews, organizes, and comments on the extensive literature on religion and coping with stress, both for younger and older adults.

**Koenig, H. G. *Is Religion Good for Your Health? The Effects of Religion on Physical and Mental Health?* New York: Haworth Press, 1997.**
Since Jeff Levin's review article in 1987 (see above), this book is the first comprehensively to review and discuss the research on religion and mental and physical health. It contains many illustrations and graphs of research findings, but in a readable format.

**Matthews, D. A. *The Faith Factor*. New York: Viking Press, 1998.**
This was the first "popular" book that discusses the research findings on religion and health and suggested clinical applications, in layperson's terms.

**Koenig, H. G., ed. *Handbook of Religion and Mental Health*. San Diego: Academic Press, 1998.**
Discusses mental health considerations when treating persons from different religious backgrounds—Christian, Muslim, Jewish, Buddhist, Hindu, and so on. Designed for the clinician, this edited collection describes how religious beliefs relate to mental health and influence mental health care. Chapters include those on religion and personality, coping behavior, anxiety, depression, psychoses, and successful psychotherapy using religious approaches.

**Koenig, H. G. *The Healing Power of Faith*. New York: Simon & Schuster, 1999.**
As with *The Faith Factor* by Dr. Matthews, above, this book is for a popular audience of general readers not very familiar with the area. Contains many inspirational stories, along with descriptions of scientific research.

**Boehnlein, J. K., ed. *Psychiatry and Religion: The Convergence of Mind and Spirit*. Washington, DC: American Psychiatric Publishing, Inc., 2000.**
This edited collection is one of the first on psychiatry and religion by the mainstream publisher, American Psychiatric Press. Focuses on religion and mental health as it applies to persons of all ages; combines research and clinical discussions.

**Koenig, H. G., M. McCullough, and D. B. Larson. *Handbook of Religion and Health*. New York: Oxford University Press, 2001.**
With over 700 pages arranged in thirty-three chapters, this text comprehensively addresses the definitions, history, research, measurement, and clinical applications for health professionals and religious professionals. An appendix contains descriptions of over 1,200 studies. Based on Google Scholar Search, no scholarly text or research article on religion and health has been cited more by researchers than the *Handbook*, which has become *the* reference text for the field of religion and health.

**Levin, J. S. *God, Faith and Health*. New York: John Wiley & Sons, 2001.**
This is Dr. Levin's popular book on religion and health. A masterful and powerful writer, Levin reviews research on religion and health and discusses its meaning for researchers and the general public.

**Koenig, H. G., and H. J. Cohen, eds.** *The Link between Religion and Health: Psychoneuroimmunology and the Faith Factor.* **New York: Oxford University Press, 2002.**
This edited volume (fifteen chapters) examines the role of psychoneuroimmunology as an explanation for the link found between religion and physical health. Leaders in psychoneuroimmunology discuss their respective areas of research and how this research can help elucidate the relationship between religion and health. This volume reviews research on religious involvement, neuroendocrine and immune function, and explores further research needed to better understand these relationships.

**Shuman, J. J., and K. G. Meador.** *Heal Thyself: Spirituality, Medicine, and the Distortion of Christianity.* **New York: Oxford University Press, 2002.**
This book critiques the research field of religion and health from a theological perspective. The authors argue convincingly that popular culture's fascination with the health benefits of religion reflects not the renaissance of the world's great religious traditions but the powerful combination of consumer capitalism and self-interested individualism. A faith-for-health exchange misrepresents and devalues the true meaning of Christian faith. They argue that such a utilitarian approach to religion may in the end not be healthy or faithful.

**Koenig, H. G.** *Faith and Mental Health: Religious Resources for Healing.* **Philadelphia: Templeton Foundation Press, 2005.**
Comprehensive and updated review of the history, research, clinical applications, and especially, the role of the church and other religious institutions in meeting the mental health needs of both their own members and those with chronic mental illness. Based on a white paper written for the Department of Health and Human Services on faith-based delivery of mental health services.

**Sloan, R. P.** *Blind Faith: The Unholy Alliance of Religion and Medicine.* **New York: St. Martin's Press, 2006.**
This book is an intensely critical review of religion and health research, religion and health researchers, and religion and health funding agencies. Discusses the author's strong ethical objections to integrating spirituality into patient care, and belief that religion and medicine should be kept completely separate.

Koenig, H. G. *Spirituality in Patient Care,* Second Edition. Philadelphia: Templeton Foundation Press, 2007.
Provides a short, practical course for health professionals of all specialties (physicians, nurses, chaplains, social workers, mental health professionals, allied-health professionals) interested in identifying and addressing the spiritual needs of patients. Included is a comprehensive curriculum for medical students and adaptations of the curriculum for nurses and other health specialists in training programs. This is a book about the whys, hows, whens, and whats of addressing spiritual issues in patient care. The second edition is completely updated, addressing concerns raised by critics over the past ten years.

Peteet, J., and F. Lu, eds. *Religion and Psychiatric Disorders for DSM-V.* Washington, DC: American Psychiatric Publishing, Inc., 2008.
Staff of the Division of Research, American Psychiatric Association, convened a panel of experts in spirituality and psychiatry to discuss how the next version of the Diagnostic and Statistical Manual (DSM-V) should be altered to address comprehensively issues related to spirituality and religion for every diagnostic category. The results of those discussions, led by John Peteet (Dana Farber Cancer Institute, Harvard) and Francis Lu (University of California at San Francisco) are published in this book, which could change the everyday practice of psychiatry.

## Internet Resources

Center for Spirituality, Theology and Health at Duke University Medical Center, Durham, North Carolina
http://www.dukespiritualityandhealth.org/

Center for Spirituality and Healing, University of Minnesota, Minneapolis
http://www.csh.umn.edu/

Center for Spirituality and Health, University of Florida, Gainesville
http://www.ufspiritualityandhealth.org/

Center for the Study of Health, Religion and Spirituality, Indiana State University, Terre Haute
http://www.indstate.edu/psych/cshrs/

**Spirituality and Health, Medical University of South Carolina, Charleston**
http://www.musc.edu/dfm/Spirituality/Spirituality.htm

**Institute for Religion and Health, Texas Medical Center, Houston**
http://www.religionandhealth.org/

**Center for Religion, the Profession, & the Public, University of Missouri, Columbia**
http://rpp.missouri.edu/D18.shtml

**George Washington Institute for Spirituality and Health, George Washington University, Washington, DC**
http://www.gwish.org/

**Center for Spirituality and the Mind, University of Pennsylvania, Philadelphia**
http://www.uphs.upenn.edu/radiology/csm/index.html

**European Research Institute for Spirituality and Health, Langenthal, Switzerland**
http://www.fisg.ch/e_html/e_support.html

**Royal College of Psychiatrists Spirituality and Psychiatry Special Interest Group, London**
http://www.rcpsych.ac.uk/college/specialinterestgroups/spirituality.aspx

**Center for Spirituality, Health and Disability, University of Aberdeen, Scotland**
http://www.abdn.ac.uk/prospectus/pgrad/study/research.php?code = spirit_health

**Association of Professional Chaplains, Schaumburg, Illinois**
http://www.professionalchaplains.org/

**International Parish Nurse Center, St. Louis**
http://www.parishnurses.org/

**David B. Larson Fellowship in Health and Spirituality, Library of Congress, Washington, DC**
http://www.loc.gov/loc/kluge/fellowships/larson.html

## AUDIO BOOKS/VIDEOS

### Audio Books

The following audio books are available from the Templeton Foundation Press at http://www.templetonpress.org

**Koenig, H. G. *Spirituality in Patient Care: Why, How, Where, and What*, First Edition. 2002.**
Discusses why and how to integrate spirituality into patient care.

**Koenig, H. G. *The Healing Connection: The Story of a Physician's Search for the Link between Faith and Health*. 2004.**
Describes Dr. Koenig's personal life story and the experiences that brought him into the field of religion, spirituality, and health. Also, discusses implications of religion-health research for the Christian community.

### Video

**"Give Me Strength: Spirituality in the Medical Encounter," developed at Johns Hopkins University.**
Discusses different definitions of spirituality, reviews studies of patient preferences regarding spirituality and health care, discusses recent research linking spirituality to improved health outcomes, and provides training for clinicians in screening and discussion of spirituality through clinical role-plays. This video is ideal for teaching student courses. Go to http://www.researchchannel.org/prog/displayevent.aspx?rID = 3110 or call 410-338-3610 to order.

## CONFERENCES

Duke University Medical Center, Durham, North Carolina
Center for Spirituality, Theology and Health
Annual National/International Conference
http://www.dukespiritualityandhealth.org/education/national.html

Mayo Clinic School of Nursing, Rochester, Minnesota
Spiritual Care Research Conference
http://www.mayoclinic.org/news2006-rst/3756.html

Harvard Medical School, Boston, Massachusetts
Spirituality and Healing in Medicine Conference
http://hssweb.net/harvard-cme/spirituality/course.htm

Johns Hopkins University, Baltimore, Maryland
Johns Hopkins Institute for Spirituality and Medicine Conference
http://www.hopkinsmedicine.org/spirituality/

Loma Linda University, Loma Linda, California
Spirituality and Health Conference
http://www.llu.edu/llu/sph/cpe/healthy/2005sh.html

Adelaide, Australia
Bi-Annual Australian Conference on Spirituality and Health
(sponsored by Adventist Health)
http://www.spiritualityhealth.org.au/

European Institute for Spirituality and Health, Bern, Switzerland
European Conference on Religion, Spirituality and Health
http://www.fisg.ch/e_html/e_events.html

## RESEARCH AND CLINICAL APPLICATIONS WORKSHOPS

**Center for Spirituality, Theology and Health**
Duke University Medical Center, Durham, North Carolina
http://www.dukespiritualityandhealth.org/education/summer-research/

**Five-day Summer Research Workshops (approved for thirty units AMA-Category I CME or CCU in previous years)**
  : intensive course involving lectures, discussions, and individual mentorship on all aspects of designing research, writing grants, execution of research projects, writing for publication, etc.

**One-day Summer Clinical Applications Workshop (continuing education credits possible)**
  : course involving lectures and discussions on how to integrate spirituality into patient care for physicians, chaplains, nurses, social workers, mental health professionals, rehabilitation specialists, and others.

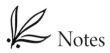 Notes

## Introduction

1. M. Angell, "Disease as a Reflection of the Psyche," *New England Journal of Medicine* 312, no. 24 (1985): 1570–72.
2. H. G. Koenig, *Spirituality in Patient Care*, 2nd ed. (Philadelphia, PA: Templeton Foundation Press, 2007).
3. H. G. Koenig, D. E. King, and K. M. Meador, *Handbook of Religion and Health*, 2nd ed. (New York: Oxford University Press, in preparation). The anticipated publication date of this volume is 2011.

## Chapter 1: Terms of the Debate

1. C. Smith and M. L. Denton, *Soul Searching: The Religious and Spiritual Lives of American Teenagers* (New York: Oxford University Press, 2005), 175.
2. A. Futterman and H. G. Koenig, "Measuring Religiosity in Later Life: What Can Gerontology Learn from the Sociology and Psychology of Religion?," background paper, published in *Proceedings of Conference on Methodological Approaches to the Study of Religion, Aging, and Health*, cosponsored by NIA and Fetzer Institute (March 16–17, 1995).
3. C. M. Puchalski, "Spirituality and Medicine: Curricula in Medical Education," *Journal of Cancer Education* 21 (2006): 14–15.
4. Association of American Medical Colleges, "Contemporary Issues in Medicine: Communication in Medicine," Medical School Objectives Project, Report III, 1999. Available at http://www.aamc.org/meded/msop/msop3.pdf (accessed January 2007).
5. G. Anandarajah and E. Hight, "Spirituality and Medical Practice: Using the HOPE Questions as a Practical Tool for Spiritual Assessment," *American Family Physician* 63 (2001): 83.
6. A. Moreira-Almeida and H. G. Koenig, "Retaining the Meaning of the Words Religiousness and Spirituality: A Commentary on the WHOQOL SRPB Group's 'A Cross-Cultural Study of Spirituality, Religion, and Personal Beliefs as Components of Quality of Life,'" *Social Science and Medicine* 63 (2006): 843–45.
7. P. C. Hill and K. I. Pargament, "Advances in the Conceptualization and Measurement of Religion and Spirituality," *American Psychologist* 58 (2003): 64–65.

8. K. I. Pargament, "The Psychology of Religion *and* Spirituality? Yes and No," *International Journal for the Psychology of Religion* 9 (1999): 12.

9. D. J. Hufford, "An Analysis of the Field of Spirituality, Religion and Health. Area I Field Analysis," 2005, http://www.metanexus.net/tarp/pdf/TARP-Hufford.pdf (last accessed January 2007).

10. Ibid.

11. Ibid.

12. H. G. Koenig, "Religion, Spirituality and Medicine in Australia: Research and Clinical Practice," *The Medical Journal of Australia* 186 (2007): S45–S46.

13. "Humanism," Wikipedia: http://en.wikipedia.org/wiki/Humanism.

14. H.G. Koenig. "Concerns About Measuring 'Spirituality' in Research." *Journal of Nervous and Mental Disease*, in press (2008).

15. H. G. Koenig, L. K. George, and P. Titus, "Religion, Spirituality and Health in Medically Ill Hospitalized Older Patients," *Journal of the American Geriatrics Association* 52 (2004): 554–62.

## CHAPTER 2: MEDICINE IN THE TWENTY-FIRST CENTURY

1. H. G. Koenig, M. M. McCullough, and D. B. Larson, *Handbook of Religion and Health* (New York: Oxford University Press, 2001), 514–89.

2. For information on the recommendations of these conferences, see: National Institute on Aging and Fetzer Institute, Conference on Methodological Approaches to the Study of Religion, Aging, and Health, Bethesda, MD, 1995; National Institute on Aging and Fetzer Institute, Working Group on Measurement of Religion/Spirituality for Healthcare Research, Bethesda, MD, 1997 (in particular, see E. L. Idler, M. A. Musick, C. G. Ellison, et al., "Measuring Multiple Dimensions of Religion and Spirituality for Health Research: Conceptual Background and Findings from the 1998 General Social Survey," *Research on Aging* 25 [2003]: 327–65); and National Institutes of Health Working Group on Spirituality, Religion, and Health, Office of Behavioral and Social Sciences Research, Bethesda, MD, 2001. This last report resulted in a special section on spirituality, religion, and health published in the January 2003 issue of the *American Psychologist* 58, no. 1.

3. W. R. Miller and C. E. Thorsen, "Spirituality, Religion and Health: An Emerging Research Field," *American Psychologist* 38 (2003): 33.

4. For questions on methodology, see R. P. Sloan, E. Bagiella, and T. Powell, "Religion, Spirituality, and Medicine," *Lancet* 353 (1999): 664–67. For a rebuttal, see H. G. Koenig, E. Idler, S. Kasl, et al., "Religion, Spirituality, and Medicine: A Rebuttal to Skeptics," *International Journal of Psychiatry in Medicine* 29 (1999): 123–31.

5. H. G. Koenig, *Spirituality in Patient Care*, 2nd ed. (Philadelphia, PA: Templeton Foundation Press, 2007).

6. Regarding these statistics, see C. M. Puchalski, "Spirituality and Medicine: Curricula in Medical Education," *Journal of Cancer Education* 21, no. 1 (2006): 14–18; and *John Templeton Foundation Capabilities Report* (West Conshohocken, PA: Templeton Foundation, 2006), 68.

7. F. A. Curlin, M. H. Chin, S. A. Sellergren, C. J. Roach, and J. D. Lantos, "The

Association of Physicians' Religious Characteristics with Their Attitudes and Self-Reported Behaviors Regarding Religion and Spirituality in the Clinical Encounter," *Medical Care* 44 (2006): 446–53.

8. See T. McNichol, "The New Faith in Medicine," *USA Weekend*, April 5–7, 1996, 5; J. Ehman, B. Ott, T. Short, R. Ciampa, and J. Hansen-Flaschen, "Do Patients Want Physicians to Inquire about Their Spiritual or Religious Beliefs If They Become Gravely Ill?" *Archives of Internal Medicine* 159 (1999): 1803–06; and D. E. King and B. Bushwick, "Beliefs and Attitudes of Hospital Inpatients about Faith Healing and Prayer," *Journal of Family Practice* 39 (1994): 349–52.

9. T. A. Balboni, L. C. Vanderwerker, S. D. Block, et al., "Religiousness and Spiritual Support among Advanced Cancer Patients and Associations with End-of-Life Treatment Preferences and Quality of Life," *Journal of Clinical Oncology* 25 (2007): 555–60.

10. K. J. Flannelly, K. Galek, and G. F. Handzo, "To What Extent Are the Spiritual Needs of Hospital Patients Being Met?" *International Journal of Psychiatry in Medicine* 35, no. 3 (2005): 319–23.

11. L. VandeCreek, "How Has Health Care Reform Affected Professional Chaplaincy Programs and How Are Department Directors Responding?" *Journal of Health Care Chaplaincy* 10, no. 1 (2000): 7–17.

12. P. A. Clark, M. Drain, and M. P. Malone, "Addressing Patients' Emotional and Spiritual Needs," *Joint Commission Journal on Quality and Safety* 29 (2003): 659–70.

13. On physicians' acknowledging the importance of spirituality, see M. R. Ellis, D. C. Vinson, and B. Ewigman, "Addressing Spiritual Concerns of Patients: Family Physicians' Attitudes and Practices," *Journal of Family Practice* 48 (1999): 105–9. On spirituality's influencing health, see H. G. Koenig, L. Bearon, and R. Dayringer, "Physician Perspectives on the Role of Religion in the Physician–Older Patient Relationship," *Journal of Family Practice* 28 (1989): 441–48; and C. A. Armbruster, J. T. Chibnall, and S. Legett, "Pediatrician Beliefs about Spirituality and Religion in Medicine: Associations with Clinical Practice," *Pediatrics* 111 (2003): E227–E235.

14. See M. H. Monroe, D. Bynum, B. Susi, et al., "Primary Care Physician Preferences Regarding Spiritual Behavior in Medical Practice," *Archives of Internal Medicine* 163 (2003): 2751–56; and T. A. Maugans and W. C. Wadland, "Religion and Family Medicine: A Survey of Physicians and Patients," *Journal of Family Practice* 32 (1991): 210–13.

15. Monroe, Bynum, Susi, et al., "Primary Care Physician Preferences Regarding Spiritual Behavior in Medical Practice."

16. J. T. Chibnall and C. A. Brooks, "Religion in the Clinic: The Role of Physician Beliefs," *Southern Medical Journal* 94 (2001): 374–79.

17. Koenig, Bearon, and Dayringer, "Physician Perspectives on the Role of Religion."

18. See Monroe, Bynum, Susi, et al., "Primary Care Physician Preferences Regarding Spiritual Behavior in Medical Practice;" and Curlin, Chin, Sellergren, Roach, and Lantos, "The Association of Physicians' Religious Characteristics . . ."

19. J. Frieden, "Incremental Changes Key to Health Care Reform," *Clinical Psychiatry News* 33, no. 4 (2005): 86.

20. "Projections of the Total Resident Population by 5-Year Age Groups, and Sex with Special Age Categories: Middle Series, 2025 to 2045," Population Projections Program, Population Division, U.S. Census Bureau, Washington, D.C. 20233. See http://www.census.gov/population/projections/nation/summary /np-t3-f.pdf.

21. "(NP-D1-A) Annual Projections of the Resident Population by Age, Sex, Race, and Hispanic Origin: High Migration Series, 1999 to 2100," Population Projections Program, Population Division, U.S. Census Bureau, Washington, D.C. 20233. See http://www.census.gov/population/projections/nation/detail/ p2041_50.c.

22. See K. Levit, C. Smith, C. Cowan, et al., "Health Spending Rebound Continues in 2002." *Health Affairs* 23, no. 1 (2004): 147–59; S. Hefler S. Smith, S. Keehan, et al., "U.S. Health Spending Projections for 2004–2014." *Health Affairs* 24, no. 1 (2005): W5/74–85; and C. Smith, C. Cowan, S. Heffler, et al. National Health Spending in 2004: Slowdown Led by Prescription Drug Spending," *Health Affairs* 25, no. 1 (2006): 186–96.

23. *Average Annual Inflation by Decade.* © 2006 InflationData.com. See http://inflationdata.com/Inflation/images/charts/Articles/Decade_inflation_chart.htm (last accessed 1/07).

24. K. Levit, C. Smith, C. Cowan, et al., "Health Spending Rebound Continues in 2002," *Health Affairs* 123, no. 1 (2004): 147–59.

25. S. Heffler, S. Smith, S. Keehan, et al., "U.S. Health Spending Projections for 2004–2014, *Health Affairs*, Web exclusive, February 23, 2005. See Web site: http://content.healthaffairs.org/cgi/reprint/hlthaff.w5.74v1 (last accessed 12/07).

26. E. L. Schneider, "Aging in the Third Millennium," *Science* 283 (1999): 796–97.

27. L. E. Hebert, P. A. Scherr, J. L. Bienias, et al., "Alzheimer Disease in the U.S. Population: Prevalence Estimates Using the 2000 Census," *Archives of Neurology* 60 (2003): 1119–22.

28. United Nations, Population Division, Department of Economic and Social Affairs, *Population Ageing—1999*, publication ST/ESA/SER.A/179.

29. P. Longman, "The Global Baby Bust," *Foreign Affairs* 83 (May/June 2004): 64–79.

30. Information taken from Wikipedia, "United States Public Debt" (September, 2006). See Web site: http://en.wikipedia.org/wiki/United_States_public_ debt#_note-0.

31. "Bernanke: Baby Boomers Threaten Economy—Fed Chief Says Failure to Deal with Aging Population Could Hurt Economy," Reuter Newswire out of Washington, D.C., reported on Cable Network News (CNN) at 12:09 p.m. on January 18, 2007.

32. These figures were calculated by dividing population age 18 or older by population age 55 or older in 2030 (301 million divided by 113 million = 38 percent). Data obtained from high series estimate for year 2030: "(NP-D1-A) Annual Projections of the Resident Population by Age, Sex, Race, and Hispanic Origin: High Migration Series, 1999 to 2100," Population Projections Program, Population Division, U.S. Census Bureau, Washington, D.C. 20233. See http://www. census.gov/population/projections/nation/detail/p2021_30.c.

33. Koenig, McCullough, and Larson, *Handbook of Religion and Health*, 24–49.
34. V. B. Carson and H. G. Koenig, *Parish Nursing* (Philadelphia: Templeton Foundation Press, 2002).
35. See D. Hale and G. Bennett, *Building Healthy Communities through Medical–Religious Partnerships* (Baltimore: Johns Hopkins University Press, 2000); and D. Hale and H. G. Koenig, *Healing Bodies, Minds and Souls: The Church's Role in Health Ministries* (Minneapolis: Fortress Press, 2003).
36. H. G. Koenig and D. Lawson, *Faith in the Future: Religion, Aging, and Healthcare in the 21st Century* (Philadelphia: Templeton Press, 2004).

CHAPTER 3: FROM MIND TO BODY

1. B. S. McEwen, "Protective and Damaging Effects of Stress Mediators," *New England Journal of Medicine* 338, no. 3 (1998): 171–79.
2. Regarding NK cell activity, see D. B. Pereira, M. H. Antoni, A. Danielson, T. Simon, et al., "Life Stress and Cervical Squamous Intraepithelial Lesions in Women with Human Papillomavirus and Human Immunodeficiency Virus," *Psychosomatic Medicine* 65, no. 3 (2003): 427–34. Regarding NK cells and cytotoxic T-cell functions, see D. Byrnes, M. H. Antoni, K. Goodkin, et al., "Stressful Events, Pessimism, Natural Killer Cell Cytotoxicity, and Cytotoxic/Suppressor T-Cells in HIV+ Black Women at Risk for Cervical Cancer," *Psychosomatic Medicine* 60 (1998): 714–22. Regarding levels of cytokines, see R. Glaser, T. Robles, J. Sheridan, W. B. Malarkey, and J. K. Kiecolt-Glaser, "Mild Depressive Symptoms Are Associated with Amplified and Prolonged Inflammatory Responses Following Influenza Vaccination in Older Adults," *Archives of General Psychiatry* 60 (2003): 1009–14.
3. On influenza virus, see Y. Deng, Y. Jing, A. E. Campbell, and S. Gravenstein, "Age-related Impaired Type 1 T Cell Responses to Influenza: Reduced Activation *Ex Vivo*, Decreased Expansion in CTL Culture *in Vitro*, and Blunted Response to Influenza Vaccination *in Vivo* in the Elderly," *Journal of Immunology* 172 (2004): 3437–46. On pneumococcal bacterium, see R. Glaser, J. F. Sheridan, W. B. Malarkey, R. C. MacCallum, and J. K. Kiecolt-Glaser, "Chronic Stress Modulates the Immune Response to a Pneumococcal Pneumonia Vaccine," *Psychosomatic Medicine* 62 (2000): 804–7. On meningococcal bacterium, see V. E. Burns, M. Drayson, C. Ring, and D. Carroll, "Perceived Stress and Psychological Well-Being Are Associated with Antibody Status after Meningitis C Conjugate Vaccination," *Psychosomatic Medicine* 64 (2002): 963–70. And for hepatitis B virus, see P. M. Jabaaij, R. A. Grosheide, and R. A. Heijtink, "Influence of Perceived Psychological Stress and Distress of Antibody Response to Low Dose rDNA Hepatitis B Vaccine," *Journal of Psychosomatic Research* 37 (1993): 361–69.
4. R. Glaser, "Stress-associated Immune Dysregulation and Its Importance for Human Health: A Personal History of Psychoneuroimmunology," *Brain, Behavior, and Immunity* 19, no. 1 (2005): 3–11.
5. See, respectively, G. Van der Pompe, M. H. Antoni, and C. Heijnen, "The Relations of Plasma ACTH and Cortisol Levels with the Distribution and Function of Peripheral Blood Cells in Response to a Behavioral Challenge in Breast Can-

cer: An Empirical Exploration by Means of Statistical Modeling," *International Journal of Behavioral Medicine* 4 (1997): 145–67; and M. Schedlowski, C. Jungk, G. Schimanski, U. Tewes, and H. J. Schmoll, "Effects of Behavioral Intervention on Plasma Cortisol and Lymphocytes in Breast Cancer Patients: An Exploratory Study," *Psycho-Oncology* 3 (1994): 181–87.

6. S. Lutgendorf, P. Vitaliano, T. Tripp-Reimer, J. Harvey, and D. Lubaroff, "Sense of Coherence Moderates the Relationship between Life Stress and Natural Killer Cell Activity in Healthy Older Adults," *Psychology and Aging* 14, no. 4 (1999): 552–63.

7. J. A. Posener, C. DeBattista, G. H. Williams, et al., "24-hour Monitoring of Cortisol and Corticotropin Secretion in Psychotic and Nonpsychotic Major Depression," *Archives of General Psychiatry* 57 (2000): 755–60.

8. J. Marx, "How the Glucocorticoids Suppress Immunity," *Science* 270 (1995): 232–33.

9. R. Glaser, L. A. Kutz, and W. B. Malarkey, "Hormonal Modulation of Epstein–Barr Virus Replication," *Neuroendocrinology* 62 (1995): 356–61.

10. R. M. Sapolsky and T. M. Donnelly, "Vulnerability to Stress-Induced Tumor Growth Increases with Age in Rats: Role of Glucocorticoids," *Endocrinology* 117 (1985): 662–66.

11. R. Glaser and J. K. Kiecolt-Glaser, "Stress-Induced Immune Dysfunction: Implications for Health," *Nature Reviews* 5 (2005): 243–51.

12. I. J. Elenkov, R. L. Wilder, G. P. Chrousos, and E. S. Vizi, "The Sympathetic Nerve—An Integrative Interface between Two Supersystems: The Brain and the Immune System," *Pharmacological Reviews* 52, no. 4 (2000): 595–638.

13. J. K. Kiecolt-Glaser, K. J. Preacher, R. C. MacCallum, et al., "Chronic Stress and Age-Related Increases in the Proinflammatory Cytokine IL-6," *Proceedings of the National Academy of Sciences* 100 (2003): 9090–95.

14. Regarding weakened immune systems, see M. Honda, K. Kitamura, Y. Mizutani, et al., "Quantitative Analysis of Serum IL-6 and Its Correlation with Increased Levels of Serum IL-2R in HIV-induced Diseases" *Journal of Immunology* 145 (1990): 4059–64. Regarding age-related immune-system cancers, see W. Ershler and E. Keller, "Age-Associated Increased Interleukin-6 Gene Expression, Late-Life Diseases, and Frailty," *Annual Review of Medicine* 51 (2000): 245–70. Regarding decline in immune function with age, see H. J. Cohen, "Editorial: In Search of the Underlying Mechanisms of Frailty," *Journal of Gerontology* 55 (2000): M706–M708.

15. K. Raikkonen, L. Keltikangas-Jarvinen, H. Adlercreutz, and A. Hautanen, "Psychosocial Stress and the Insulin Resistance Syndrome," *Metabolism* 45 (1996): 1533–38.

16. J. Zhang, R. Niaura, J. R. Dyer, et al., "Hostility and Urine Norepinephrine Interact to Predict Insulin Resistance: The VA Normative Aging Study," *Psychosomatic Medicine* 68 (2006): 718–26.

17. S. Melamed, A. Shirom, S. Toker, and I. Shapira, "Burnout and Risk of Type II Diabetes: A Prospective Study of Apparently Healthy Employed Persons," *Psychosomatic Medicine* 68, no. 6 (2006): 863–69.

18. P. S. Eriksson and L. Wallin, "Functional Consequences of Stress-Related Suppression of Adult Hippocampal Neurogenesis—A Novel Hypothesis on

the Neurobiology of Burnout," *Acta Neurologica Scandinavica* 110 (2004): 275–80.

19. R. S. Wilson, S. E. Arnold, J. A. Schneider, Y. Li, and D. A. Bennett, "Chronic Distress, Age-Related Neuropathology, and Late-Life Dementia," *Psychosomatic Medicine* 69 (2007): 47–53.

20. L. A. Pratt, D. E. Ford, R. M. Crum, H. K. Armenian, J. J. Gallo, and W. W. Eaton, "Depression, Psychotropic Medication, and Risk of Myocardial Infarction. Prospective Data from the Baltimore ECA Follow-Up," *Circulation* 94 (1996): 3123–29.

21. J. A. Blumenthal, H. S. Lett, M. A. Babyak, et al., for the NORG Investigators, "Depression as a Risk Factor for Mortality after Coronary Artery Bypass Surgery," *Lancet* 362 (2003): 604–9.

22. R. Schulz and S. R. Beach, "Caregiving as a Risk Factor for Mortality: The Caregiver Health Effects Study," *Journal of the American Medical Association* 282 (1999): 2215–19.

23. S. Lee, G. A. Colditz, L. F. Berkman, and I. Kawachi, "Caregiving and Risk of Coronary Heart Disease in U.S. Women: A Prospective Study," *American Journal of Preventative Medicine* 24 (2003): 113–19.

24. S. Lee, G. Colditz, L. Berkman, and I. Kawachi, "Caregiving to Children and Grandchildren and Risk of Coronary Heart Disease in Women," *American Journal of Public Health* 93 (2003): 1939–44.

25. T. Q. Miller, T. W. Smith, C. W. Turner, M. L. Guijarro, and A. J. Hallet, "A Meta-analytic Review of Research on Hostility and Physical Health," *Psychological Bulletin* 119 (1996): 322–48.

26. I. Kawachi, D. Sparrow, A. I. Spiro, P. Vokonas, and S. T. Weiss, "A Prospective Study of Anger and Coronary Heart Disease: The Normative Aging Study," *Circulation* 84 (1995): 2090–95.

27. C. Iribarren, S. Sidney, D. E. Bild, K. Liu, J. H. Markovitz, et al., "Association of Hostility with Coronary Artery Calcification in Young Adults—The CARDIA Study," *Journal of the American Medical Association* 283 (2000): 2546–51.

28. W. Jiang, J. Alexander, E. Christopher, et al., "Relationship of Depression to Increased Risk of Mortality and Rehospitalization in Patients with Congestive Heart Failure," *Archives of Internal Medicine* 161 (2001): 1849–56.

29. M. D. Sullivan, W. C. Levy, B. A. Crane, J. E. Russo, and J. A. Spertus, "Usefulness of Depression to Predict Time to Combined End Point of Transplant or Death for Outpatients with Advanced Heart Failure," *American Journal of Cardiology* 94, no. 12 (2004): 1577–80.

30. E. E. Ming, G. K. Adler, R. C. Kessler, et al., "Cardiovascular Reactivity to Work Stress Predicts Subsequent Onset of Hypertension: The Air Traffic Controller Health Change Study," *Psychosomatic Medicine* 66, no. 4 (2004): 459–65.

31. K. Davidson, B. S. Jonas, K. E. Dixon, and J. H. Markovitz, "Do Depression Symptoms Predict Early Hypertension Incidence in Young Adults in the CARDIA Study? Coronary Artery Risk Development in Young Adults," *Archives of Internal Medicine* 160 (2000):1495–1500.

32. L. L. Yan, K. Liu, K. A. Matthews, et al., "Psychosocial Factors and Risk of Hypertension: The Coronary Artery Risk Development in Young Adults (CARDIA) Study," *Journal of the American Medical Association* 290 (2003): 2138–48.

33. B. B. Gump, K. A. Matthews, L. E. Eberly, Y. F. Chang, and M. R. Group, "Depressive Symptoms and Mortality in Men: Results from the Multiple Risk Factor Intervention Trial," *Stroke* 36, no. 1 (2005): 98–102.

34. S. C. Lewis, M. S. Dennis, S. J. O'Rourke, and M. Sharpe, "Negative Attitudes among Short-Term Stroke Survivors Predict Worse Long-Term Survival," *Stroke* 32 (2001): 1640–45.

35. B. T. Baune, I. Adrian, V. Arolt, and K. Berger, "Associations between Major Depression, Bipolar Disorders, Dysthymia and Cardiovascular Diseases in the General Adult Population," *Psychotherapy & Psychosomatics* 75, no. 5 (2006): 319–26.

36. See S. Cohen, D. A. Tyrrell, and A. P. Smith, "Psychological Stress and Susceptibility to the Common Cold," *New England Journal of Medicine* 325 (1991): 606–12; and S. Cohen, E. Frank, W. J. Doyle, et al., "Types of Stressors That Increase Susceptibility to the Common Cold in Healthy Adults," *Health Psychology* 17 (1998): 214–23.

37. A. A. Stone, D.H. Bovbjerg, J. M. Neale, et al., "Development of Common Cold Symptoms Following Experimental Rhinovirus Infection Is Related to Prior Stressful Life Events," *Behavioral Medicine* 18 (1992): 115–20.

38. Cohen, Frank, Doyle, et al., "Types of Stressors That Increase Susceptibility to the Common Cold in Healthy Adults."

39. S. A. Plotkin, "Immunologic Correlates of Protection Induced by Vaccination," *Pediatric Infectious Disease* 20 (2001): 73–75.

40. S. Werner and R. Grose, "Regulation of Wound Healing by Growth Factors and Cytokines," *Physiology Reviews* 83 (2003): 835–70.

41. Concerning mice, see D. A. Padgett, P. T. Marucha, and J. F. Sheridan, "Restraint Stress Slows Cutaneous Wound Healing in Mice," *Brain, Behavior, and Immunity* 12 (1998): 64–73. Concerning stressed students during exam week, see P. T. Marucha, J. K. Kiecolt-Glaser, and M. Favagehi, "Mucosal Wound Healing Is Impaired by Examinations Stress," *Psychosomatic Medicine* 60 (1998): 362–65. Regarding marital stress, see J. K. Kiecolt-Glaser, T. J. P. Loving, J. R. P. Stowell JRP, et al., "Hostile Marital Interactions, Proinflammatory Cytokine Production, and Wound Healing," *Archives of General Psychiatry* 62, no. 12 (2005): 1377–84. For study on elective surgery patients, see L. McGuire, K. Heffner, R. Glaser, et al., "Pain and Wound Healing in Surgical Patients," *Annals of Behavioral Medicine* 31, no. 2 (2006): 165–72. Finally, concerning stress among caregivers, see J. K. Kiecolt-Glaser, P. T. Marucha, W. B. Malarkey, A. M. Mercado, and R. Glaser, "Slowing of Wound Healing by Psychological Stress," *Lancet* 346, no. 8984 (1996): 1194–96.

42. J. E. Graham, L. M. Christian, and J. K. Kiecolt-Glaser, "Stress, Age, and Immune Function: Toward a Lifespan Approach," *Journal of Behavioral Medicine* 29, no. 4 (2006): 389–400.

43. I. Rojas, D. A. Padgett, J. F. Sheridan, and P. T. Marucha, "Stress-induced Susceptibility to Bacterial Infection during Cutaneous Wound Healing," *Brain, Behavior, and Immunity* 16 (2002): 74–84.

44. K. W. Brown, A. R. Levy, Z. Rosberger, and L. Edgar, "Psychological Distress and Cancer Survival: A Follow-Up 10 Years after Diagnosis," *Psychosomatic Medicine* 65 (2003): 636–43.

45. I. Levav, R. Kohn, J. Iscovich, et al., "Cancer Incidence and Survival Following Bereavement," *American Journal of Public Health* 90 (2000): 1601–7.

46. See the following: S. Greer, T. Morris, and K. W. Pettingale, "Psychological Response to Breast Cancer: Effect on Outcome," *Lancet* 2 (1979): 785–87; S. Greer, T. Morris, K. W. Pettingale, and J. L. Haybittle, "Psychological Response to Breast Cancer and 15-Year Outcome," *Lancet* 335 (1990): 49–50; and M. Watson, J. S. Haviland, S. Greer, J. Davidson, and J. M. Bliss, "Influence of Psychological Response on Survival in Breast Cancer," *Lancet* 354 (1999): 1331–36.

47. S. Mallik, H. M. Krumholz, Z. Q. Lin, et al., "Patients with Depressive Symptoms Have Lower Health Status Benefits after Coronary Artery Bypass Surgery," *Circulation* 111, no. 3 (2005): 271–77.

48. S. Cohen and T. A. Wills, "Stress, Social Support, and the Buffering Hypothesis," *Psychological Bulletin* 98, no. 2 (1985): 310–57.

49. See J. K. Kiecolt-Glaser, W. Garner, C. Speicher, et al., "Psychosocial Modifiers of Immunocompetence in Medical Students," *Psychosomatic Medicine* 46 (1984): 7–14; and J. K. Kiecolt-Glaser, R. Glaser, E. C. Strain, et al., "Modulation of Cellular Immunity in Medical Students," *Journal of Behavioral Medicine* 9 (1986): 311–20.

50. A. Picardi, F. Battisti, L. Tarsitani, et al., "Attachment Security and Immunity in Healthy Women," *Psychosomatic Medicine* 69 (2007): 40–46.

51. See R. M. Sapolsky, "The Influence of Social Hierarchy on Primate Health," *Science* 308, no. 5722 (2005): 648–52; and M. M. Sanchez, F. Aguado, F. Sanchez-Toscano, and D. Saphier, "Effects of Prolonged Social Isolation on Responses of Neurons in the Bed Nucleus of the Stria Terminalis, Preoptic Area, and Hypothalamic Paraventricular Nucleus to Stimulation of the Medial Amygdale," *Psychoneuroendocrinology* 20 (1995): 525–41.

52. M. C. Rosal, J. King, Y. Ma, and G. W. Reed, "Stress, Social Support, and Cortisol: Inverse Associations?" *Behavioral Medicine* 30, no. 1 (2004): 11–21.

53. N. Kawakami, K. Akachi, H. Shimizu, et al., "Job Strain, Social Support in the Workplace, and Haemoglobin A1c in Japanese Men," *Occupational and Environmental Medicine* 57 (2000): 805–9.

54. B. M. van Gelder, M. Tijhuis, S. Kalmijn, S. Giampaoli, A. Nissinen, and D. Kromhout, "Marital Status and Living Situation during a 5-Year Period Are Associated with a Subsequent 10-Year Cognitive Decline in Older Men: The FINE Study," *Journals of Gerontology Series B: Psychological Sciences and Social Sciences* 61, no. 4 (2006): P213–P219.

55. R. M. Sapolsky, "Glucocorticoids and Hippocampal Atrophy in Neuropsychiatric Disorders," *Archives of General Psychiatry* 57, no. 10 (2000): 925–35.

56. H. Hemingway and M. Marmot, "Evidence Based Cardiology: Psychosocial Factors in the Aetiology and Prognosis of Coronary Heart Disease. Systematic Review of Prospective Cohort Studies," *British Medical Journal* 318 (1999): 1460–67.

57. B. H. Brummett, J. C. Barefoot, I. C. Siegler, et al., "Characteristics of Socially Isolated Patients with Coronary Artery Disease Who Are at Elevated Risk for Mortality," *Psychosomatic Medicine* 63 (2001): 267–72.

58. P. M. Eng, E. B. Rimm, G. Fitzmaurice, and I. Kawachi, "Social Ties and Change in Social Ties in Relation to Subsequent Total and Cause-Specific Mortality and

Coronary Heart Disease Incidence in Men," *American Journal of Epidemiology* 155 (2002): 700–9.

59. See J. S. Goodwin, W. C. Hunt, C. R. Key, and J. M. Samet, "The Effect of Marital Status on Stage, Treatment, and Survival of Cancer Patients," *Journal of the American Medical Association* 258 (1987): 3125–30; and J. S. House, K. R. Landis, and D. Umberson, "Social Relationships and Health," *Science* 241 (1988): 540–45.

60. M. A. Price, C. C. Tennant, P. N. Butow, et al., "The Role of Psychosocial Factors in the Development of Breast Carcinoma: Part II," *Cancer* 91 (2001): 686–97.

61. S. K. Lutgendorf, "Individual Differences and Immune Function: Implications for Cancer," *Brain, Behavior, and Immunity* 17 (2003) (suppl 1): S106–S108.

62. S. K. Lutgendorf, E. Johnsen, R. Holmes, et al., "Social Relationships and Tumor Angiogenesis Factors in Ovarian Cancer Patients," *Cancer* 95 (2002): 808–15.

63. See R. Glaser and J. K. Kiecolt-Glaser, "Stress-induced Immune Dysfunction: Implications for Health," *Nature Reviews* 5 (2005): 243–51; and S. C. Segerstrom, "Individual Differences, Immunity, and Cancer: Lessons from Personality Psychology," *Brain, Behavior, and Immunity* 17 (2003) (suppl. 1): S92–S97.

64. Regarding animal studies, see L. D. Caren, J. A Leveque, and A. D. Mandel, "Effect of Ethanol on the Immune System in Mice," *Developments in Toxicology and Environmental Science* 11 (1983): 435–38. On human studies, see J. Lundy, J. H. Raaf, S. Deakins, et al., "The Acute and Chronic Effects of Alcohol on the Human Immune System," *Surgery, Gynecology & Obstetrics* 141 (1975): 212–18; and R. R. MacGregor, "Alcohol and Immune Defense," *Journal of the American Medical Association* 256 (1986): 1474–79.

65. See Lundy, Raaf, Deakins, et al., "The Acute and Chronic Effects of Alcohol on the Human Immune System."

66. P. G. Holt, "Immune and Inflammatory Function in Cigarette Smokers," *Thorax* 42 (1987): 241–49.

67. C. J. Meliska, M. E. Strunkard, D. J. Gilbert, R. A. Jensen, and J. M. Martinko, "Immune Function in Cigarette Smokers Who Quit Smoking for 31 Days," *Journal of Allergy and Clinical Immunology* 95 (1995): 901–10.

68. W. Jung and M. Irwin, "Reduction of Natural Killer Cytotoxic Activity in Major Depression: Interaction between Depression and Cigarette Smoking," *Psychosomatic Medicine* 61 (1999): 263–70.

69. See L. Ferrucci, T. Harris, J. Guralnik, et al., "Serum IL-6 Level and the Development of Disability in Older Persons," *Journal of the American Geriatrics Society* 47 (1999):639–46; and D. R. Taaffe, T. B. Harris, L. Ferrucci, et al., "Crosssectional and Prospective Relationships of Interleukin-6 and C-Reactive Protein with Physical Performance in Elderly Persons: MacArthur Studies of Successful Aging," *Journal of Gerontology Series A: Biological Sciences and Medical Sciences* 55 (2000): M709–M715.

70. See R. F. Anda, D. F. Williamson, L. G. Escobedo, E. E. Mast, G. A. Giovino, and P. L. Remington, "Depression and the Dynamics of Smoking: A National Perspective," *Journal of the American Medical Association* 264 (1990): 1541–45; and D. D. Lobstein, B. J. Mosbacher, and A. H. Ismail, "Depression as a Powerful

Discriminator between Physically Active and Sedentary Middle-aged Men," *Journal of Psychosomatic Research* 27 (1983): 69–76.

71. F. Bonnet, K. Irving, J. L. Terra, P. Nony, F. Berthezene, and P. Moulin, "Anxiety and Depression Are Associated with Unhealthy Lifestyle in Patients at Risk of Cardiovascular Disease," *Atherosclerosis* 178, no. 2 (2005): 339–44.

72. K. I. Hunter and M. W. Linn, "Psychosocial Differences between Elderly Volunteers and Non-Volunteers," *International Journal of Aging in Human Development* 12 (1980–81): 205–13.

73. C. Schwartz, J. B. Beisenhelder, M. Yunsheng, and G. Reed, "Altruistic Social Interest Behaviors Are Associated with Better Mental Health," *Psychosomatic Medicine* 65 (2003): 778–85.

74. See N. Morrow-Howell, J. Hinterlong, P. A. Rozario, and F. Tang, "Effects of Volunteering on the Well-Being of Older Adults," *Journals of Gerontology Series B: Psychological Sciences and Social Sciences* 58, no. 3 (2003): S137–S145; J. Liang, N. M. Krause, and J. M. Bennett, "Social Exchange and Well-Being: Is Giving Better Than Receiving?" *Psychology & Aging* 16, no. 3 (2001): 511–23; H. K. Yuen, "Impact of an Altruistic Activity on Life Satisfaction in Institutionalized Elders: A Pilot Study," *Physical & Occupational Therapy in Geriatrics* 20, nos. 3–4 (2002): 125–35; M. A. Musick and J. Wilson, "Volunteering and Depression: The Role of Psychological and Social Resources in Different Age Groups," *Social Science & Medicine* 56, no. 2 (2003): 259–69; P. Dulin and R. Hill, "Relationships between Altruistic Activity and Positive and Negative Affect among Low-Income Older Adult Service Providers," *Aging & Mental Health* 7, no. 4 (2003): 294–99; and R. F. Krueger, B. M. Hicks, and M. McGue, "Altruism and Antisocial Behavior: Independent Tendencies, Unique Personality Correlates, Distinct Etiologies," *Psychological Science* 12, no. 5 (2001): 397–402.

75. S. L. Brown, R. M. Nesse, A. D. Vinokur, and D. M. Smith, "Providing Social Support May Be More Beneficial Than Receiving It: Results from a Prospective Study of Mortality," *Psychological Science* 14, no. 4 (2003): 320–27.

76. D. Oman, C. E. Thoresen, K. McMahon, "Volunteerism and Mortality among the Community-Dwelling Elderly," *Journal of Health Psychology* 4 (1999): 301–16.

77. J. Moll, F. Krueger, R. Zahn, M. Pardini, R. de Oliveira-Souza, and J. Grafman, "Human Fronto-mesolimbic Networks Guide Decisions about Charitable Donation," *Proceedings of the National Academy of Sciences* 103, no. 42 (2006): 15623–28.

78. A. A. Carlson, A. F. Russell, A. J. Young, et al., "Elevated Prolactin Levels Immediately Precede Decisions to Babysit by Male Meerkat Helpers," *Hormones & Behavior* 50, no. 1 (2006): 94–100.

79. S. J. Schoech, "Physiology of Helping in Florida Scrub-Jays," in *Exploring Animal Behavior: Readings from American Scientist*, 4th ed., ed. P. W. Sherman and J. Alcock, 117–24 (Sunderland, MA: Sinauer Associates, 2005).

80. See A. Luks, "Helper's High: Volunteering Makes People Feel Good, Physically and Emotionally. And Like 'Runner's Calm,' It's Probably Good For Your Health," *Psychology Today* (October 1988): 39, 42.

81. G. B. Stefano, G. L. Fricchione, B. T. Glingsby, and H. Benson, "The Placebo Effect and Relaxation Response: Neural Processes and Their Coupling to Constitutive Nitric Oxide," *Brain Research Reviews* 35 (2001): 1–19.

CHAPTER 4: RELIGION AND HEALTH

1. H. G. Koenig, M. E. McCullough, and D. B. Larson, *Handbook of Religion and Health* (New York: Oxford University Press, 2001).

2. M. A. Schuster, B. D. Stein, L. H. Jaycox, "A National Survey of Stress Reactions after the September 11, 2001, Terrorist Attacks," *New England Journal of Medicine* 345 (2001): 1507–12.

3. H. G. Koenig, "Religious Beliefs and Practices of Hospitalized Medically Ill Older Adults," *International Journal of Geriatric Psychiatry* 13 (1998): 213–24.

4. H. G. Koenig, L. K. George, and P. Titus, "Religion, Spirituality and Health in Medically Ill Hospitalized Older Patients," *Journal of the American Geriatrics Association* 52 (2004): 554–62.

5. T. A. Cronan, R. M. Kaplan, L. Posner, E. Lumberg, and F. Kozin, "Prevalence of the Use of Unconventional Remedies for Arthritis in a Metropolitan Community," *Arthritis and Rheumatism* 32 (1989): 1604–7.

6. L. Tepper, S. A. Rogers, E. M. Coleman, et al. "The Prevalence of Religious Coping among Persons with Persistent Mental Illness," *Psychiatric Services* 52, no. 5 (2001): 660–65.

7. A. Rammohan, K. Rao, D. K. Subbakrishna, "Religious Coping and Psychological Wellbeing in Carers of Relatives with Schizophrenia," *Acta Psychiatrica Scandinavica* 105, no. 5 (2002): 356–62.

8. A. Kesselring, M. J. Dodd, A. M. Lindsey, and A. L. Strauss, "Attitudes of Patients Living in Switzerland about Cancer and Its Treatment," *Cancer Nursing* 9 (1986): 77–85.

9. R. D'Souza, "Do Patients Expect Psychiatrists to Be Interested in Spiritual Issues?" *Australasian Psychiatry* 10, no. 1 (2002): 44–47.

10. Koenig, McCullough, and Larson, *Handbook of Religion and Health*, 525–26.

11. S. J. Cutler, "Membership in Different Types of Voluntary Associations and Psychological Well-Being," *The Gerontologist* 16 (1976): 335–39.

12. N. Krause, "Exploring the Stress-Buffering Effects of Church-based and Secular Social Support on Self-Rated Health in Late Life," *Journals of Gerontology Series B: Psychological Sciences and Social Sciences* 61, no. 1 (2006): S35–S43.

13. See J. M. Salsman, T. L. Brown, E. H. Brechting, C. R. Carlson, "The Link between Religion and Spirituality and Psychological Adjustment: The Mediating Role of Optimism and Social Support," *Personality & Social Psychology Bulletin* 31, no. 4 (2005): 522–35; and C. G. Watlington and C. M. Murphy, "The Roles of Religion and Spirituality among African American Survivors of Domestic Violence," *Journal of Clinical Psychology* 62, no. 7 (2006): 837–57.

14. H. G. Koenig, D. O. Moberg, and J. N. Kvale, "Religious Activities and Attitudes of Older Adults in a Geriatric Assessment Clinic," *Journal of the American Geriatrics Society* 36 (1988): 362–74.

15. J. M. Wallace and T. A. Forman, "Religion's Role in Promoting Health and Reducing the Risk among American Youth," *Health Education and Behavior* 25 (1998): 721–41.

16. Koenig, McCullough, and Larson, *Handbook of Religion and Health*. See 181–90, 218–19, and 545–46.

17. R. Stark, "Religion as Context: Hellfire and Delinquency One More Time," *Sociology of Religion* 57 (1996): 163–73.

18. B. R. Johnson, *The Great Escape: How Religion Alters the Delinquent Behavior of High-Risk Adolescents* (Philadelphia: Center for Research on Religion and Urban Civil Society, University of Pennsylvania, 2003).

19. B. R. Johnson, *The InnerChange Freedom Initiative: A Preliminary Evaluation of a Faith-Based Prison Program* (Philadelphia: Center for Research on Religion and Urban Civil Society, University of Pennsylvania, 2003).

20. T. I. Herrenkohl, E. A. Tajima, S. D. Whitney, and B. Huang, "Protection against Antisocial Behavior in Children Exposed to Physically Abusive Discipline," *Journal of Adolescent Health* 36, no. 6 (2005): 457–65.

21. E. Hausmann, "Chaplain Contacts Improve Treatment Outcomes in Residential Treatment Programs for Delinquent Adolescents," *Journal of Pastoral Care & Counseling* 58, no. 3 (2004): 215–24.

22. C. O. Butts III, G. B. Stefano, G. Fricchione, and E. Salamon, "Religion and Its Effects on Crime and Delinquency," *Medical Science Monitor* 9, no. 8 (2003): SR79–SR82.

23. "CASA Report: Spirituality and Religion Reduce Risk of Substance Abuse." See http://www.casacolumbia.org/absolutenm/templates/PressReleases.asp?articleid=115&zoneid=48 (last accessed 3/3/07).

24. Koenig, McCullough, and Larson, *Handbook of Religion and Health*. See 539–43.

25. See S. Sussman, S. Skara, Y. Rodriguez, and P. Pokhrel, "Non Drug Use– and Drug Use–Specific Spirituality As One-Year Predictors of Drug Use among High-Risk Youth," *Substance Use & Misuse* 41, no. 13 (2006): 1801–16; and M. A. Collins, "Religiousness and Spirituality as Possible Recovery Variables in Treated and Natural Recoveries: A Qualitative Study," *Alcoholism Treatment Quarterly* 24, no. 4 (2007): 119–35.

26. For a study on Native Americans, see R. A. Stone, L. B. Whitbeck, X. Chen, K. Johnson, and D. M. Olson, "Traditional Practices, Traditional Spirituality, and Alcohol Cessation among American Indians," *Journal of Studies on Alcohol* 67, no. 2 (2006): 236–44. Regarding Hispanics, see F. F. Marsiglia, S. Kulis, T. Nieri, and M. Parsai, "God Forbid! Substance Use among Religious and Non-Religious Youth," *American Journal of Orthopsychiatry* 75, no. 4 (2005): 585–98. Concerning African Americans, see A. Nasim, S. O. Utsey, R. Corona, and F. Z. Belgrade, "Religiosity, Refusal Efficacy, and Substance Use among African-American Adolescents and Young Adults," *Journal of Ethnicity in Substance Abuse* 5, no. 3 (2006): 29–49; and K. J. Steinman and M. A. Zimmerman, "Religious Activity and Risk Behavior among African American Adolescents: Concurrent and Developmental Effects," *American Journal of Community Psychology* 33, nos. 3–4 (2004): 151–61.

27. Koenig, McCullough, and Larson, *Handbook of Religion and Health*, 543–45.

28. Sussman, Skara, Rodriguez, and Pokhrel, "Non Drug Use– and Drug Use–Specific Spirituality . . ."

29. H. R. White, B. J. McMorris, R. F. Catalano, et al., "Increases in Alcohol and Marijuana Use during the Transition Out of High School into Emerging Adulthood: The Effects of Leaving Home, Going to College, and High School Protective Factors," *Journal of Studies on Alcohol* 67, no. 6 (2006): 810–22.

30. Steinman and Zimmerman, "Religious Activity and Risk Behavior among African American Adolescents."

31. S. M. Kogan, Z. Luo, V. M. Murry, and G. H. Brody, "Risk and Protective Factors for Substance Use among African American High School Dropouts," *Psychology and Addiction Behavior* 19, no. 4 (2005): 382–91.

32. D. R. Brown, W. Scott, K. Lacey, et al., "Black Churches in Substance Use and Abuse Prevention Efforts," *Journal of Alcohol and Drug Education* 50, no. 2 (2006): 43–65.

33. See M. Galanter, "Innovations: Alcohol and Drug Abuse: Spirituality in Alcoholics Anonymous: A Valuable Adjunct to Psychiatric Services," *Psychiatric Services* 57, no. 3 (2006): 307–9; W. R. Miller and K. M. Carroll, *Rethinking Substance Abuse: What the Science Shows, and What We Should Do about It* (New York: Guilford Press, 2006); and M. Sharma, "Editorial: Religiosity and Substance Abuse: Need for Systematic Research," *Journal of Alcohol and Drug Education* 50, no. 1 (2006): 1–4.

34. Koenig, McCullough, and Larson, *Handbook of Religion and Health*, 547–48.

35. See S. M. Myers, "Religious Homogamy and Marital Quality: Historical and Generational Patterns, 1980–1997," *Journal of Marriage and Family* 68, no. 2 (2006): 292–304; S. P. Martin and S. Parashar, "Women's Changing Attitudes toward Divorce, 1974–2002: Evidence for an Educational Crossover," *Journal of Marriage and Family* 68, no. 1 (2006): 29–40; and O. S. Hunler and T. Gencoz, "The Effect of Religiousness on Marital Satisfaction: Testing the Mediator Role of Marital Problem Solving between Religiousness and Marital Satisfaction Relationship," *Contemporary Family Therapy* 27, no. 1 (2005): 123–36.

36. Martin and Parashar, "Women's Changing Attitudes toward Divorce, 1974–2002."

37. Hunler and Gencoz, "The Effect of Religiousness on Marital Satisfaction."

38. L. C. Mullins, K. P. Brackett, D. W. Bogie, and D. Pruett, "The Impact of Religious Homogeneity on Divorce in the United States," *Sociological Inquiry* 74 (2004): 338–54.

39. L. C. Mullins, K. P. Brackett, D. W. Bogie, and D. Pruett, "The Impact of Concentrations of Religious Denominational Affiliations on the Rate of Currently Divorced in Counties in the United States," *Journal of Family Issues* 27, no. 7 (2006): 976–1000.

40. Koenig, McCullough, and Larson, *Handbook of Religion and Health*, 571–72.

41. See C. Odimegwu, "Influence of Religion on Adolescent Sexual Attitudes and Behaviour among Nigerian University Students: Affiliation or Commitment?" *African Journal of Reproductive Health* 9, no. 2 (2005): 125–40; D. W. Holder, R. H. Durant, T. L. Harris, J. H. Daniel, D. Obeidallah, and E. Goodman, "The Association between Adolescent Spirituality and Voluntary Sexual Activity," *Journal of Adolescent Health* 26, no. 4 (2000): 295–302; M. Mouttapa, T. T. Huang, S. Shakib, S. Sussman, and J. B. Unger, "Authority-related Conformity as a Protective Factor against Adolescent Health Risk Behaviors," *Journal of Adolescent Health* 33, no. 5 (2003): 320–21; J. Ball, L. Armistead, and B. J. Austin, "The Relationship between Religiosity and Adjustment among African-American, Female, Urban Adolescents," *Journal of Adolescence* 26, no. 4 (2003): 431–46; and C. Paul, J. Fitzjohn, J. Eberhart-Phillips, P. Herbison, and N. Dickson, "Sexual Abstinence at Age 21 in New Zealand: The Importance of Reli-

gion," *Social Science & Medicine* 51, no. 1 (2000): 1–10.

42. S. Folkman, M. A. Chesney, L. Pollack, and C. Phillips, "Stress, Coping, and High-Risk Sexual Behavior," *Health Psychology* 11 (1992): 218–22.

43. See R. K. Jones, J. E. Darroch, and S. Singh, "Religious Differentials in the Sexual and Reproductive Behaviors of Young Women in the United States," *Journal of Adolescent Health* 36, no. 4 (2005): 279–88; and L. Miller and M. Gur, "Religiousness and Sexual Responsibility in Adolescent Girls," *Journal of Adolescent Health* 31, no. 5 (2002): 401–6.

44. M. W. Ross and M. E. Fernandez-Esquer, "Ethnicity in Sexually Transmitted Infections and Sexual Behaviour Research," *Lancet* 365, no. 9466 (2005): 1209–10.

45. S. M. Naguib, G. W. Comstock, and H. J. Davis, "Epidemiologic Study of Trichomoniasis in Normal Women," *Obstetrics and Gynecology* 27 (1966): 607–16.

46. See R. L. Stoneburner and D. Low-Beer, "Population-level HIV Declines and Behavioral Risk Avoidance in Uganda," *Science* 304 (2004): 714–18; and J. D. Shelton, D. T. Halperin, V. Nantulya, et al., "Partner Reduction Is Crucial for Balanced 'ABC' Approach to HIV Prevention," *British Medical Journal* 328 (2004): 891–93.

47. See S. N. Seidman, W. D. Mosher, and S. O. Aral, "Women with Multiple Sexual Partners: United States, 1988." *American Journal of Public Health* 82 (1992): 1388–94; J. O. G. Billy, K. Tanfer, W. R. Grady, and D. H. Klepinger, "The Sexual Behavior of Men in the United States," *Family Planning Perspectives* 25, no. 2 (1993): 52–60; and L. Nicholas and K. Durrheim, "Religiosity, AIDS, and Sexuality Knowledge, Attitudes, Beliefs, and Practices of Black South-African First-Year University Students," *Psychological Reports* 77 (1995): 1328–30.

48. P. B. Gray, "HIV and Islam: Is HIV Prevalence Lower among Muslims?" *Social Science & Medicine* 58, no. 9 (2004): 1751–56.

49. C. A. Ford, B. W. Pence, W. C. Miller, et al., "Predicting Adolescents' Longitudinal Risk for Sexually Transmitted Infection: Results from the National Longitudinal Study of Adolescent Health," *Archives of Pediatrics & Adolescent Medicine* 159, no. 7 (2005): 657–64.

50. See M. A. Musick, A. R. Herzog, and J. S. House, "Volunteering and Mortality among Older Adults: Findings from a National Sample," *Journals of Gerontology Series B: Psychological Sciences and Social Sciences* 54B, no. 3 (1999): S173–S180; and V. Hodgkinson and R. Wuthnow, *Faith and Philanthropy in America* (San Francisco: Jossey-Bass, 1990).

51. J. Z. Park and C. Smith. "'To Whom Much Has Been Given . . .': Religious Capital and Community Voluntarism among Churchgoing Protestants," *Journal for the Scientific Study of Religion* 39 (2000): 272–86.

52. Independent Sector: About Us. See http://www.independentsector.org/about /index.html (last accessed 3/5/07).

53. Independent Sector, "Giving and Volunteering in the United States: Key Findings," 2001. See http://www.independentsector.org/PDFs/GV01keyfind.pdf (last accessed 3/5/07).

54. Ibid., "The New Non-Profit Almanac in Brief: Facts and Figures on the Independent Sector," 2001.

55. C. Schwartz, J. B. Meisenhelder, Y. Ma, and G. Reed, "Altruistic Social Interest

Behaviors Are Associated with Better Mental Health," *Psychosomatic Medicine* 65, no. 5 (2003): 778–85.

56. C. D. Batson, P. Schoenrade, and W. L. Ventis, *Religion and the Individual: A Social-Psychological Perspective* (New York: Oxford University Press, 1993).

57. V. Saroglou, I. Pichon, L. Trompette, M. Verschueren, and R. Dernelle, "Prosocial Behavior and Religion: New Evidence Based on Projective Measures and Peer Ratings," *Journal for the Scientific Study of Religion* 44, no. 3 (2005): 323–48.

## CHAPTER 5: MENTAL HEALTH

1. S. B. Guze and E. Robins, "Suicide in Primary Affective Disorders, *British Journal of Psychiatry* 117 (1970): 437–38.

2. H. G. Koenig, L. K. George, B. L. Peterson, and C. F. Pieper, "Depression in Medically Ill Hospitalized Older Adults: Prevalence, Correlates, and Course of Symptoms Based on Six Diagnostic Schemes," *American Journal of Psychiatry* 154 (1997): 1376–83.

3. H. G. Koenig and D. G. Blazer, "Epidemiology of Geriatric Depression," *Clinics in Geriatric Medicine* 8, no. 2 (1992): 235–51.

4. H. G. Koenig, F. Shelp, V. Goli, H. J. Cohen, and D. G. Blazer, "Survival and Healthcare Utilization in Elderly Medical Inpatients with Major Depression," *Journal of the American Geriatrics Society* 37 (1989): 599–606.

5. H. G. Koenig, M. E. McCullough, and D. B. Larson, *Handbook of Religion and Health* (New York: Oxford University Press, 2001), 527–30.

6. Ibid., 531–35.

7. T. B. Smith, M. E. McCullough, and J. Poll, "Religiousness and Depression: Evidence for a Main Effect and the Moderating Influence of Stressful Life Events," *Psychological Bulletin* 129, no. 4 (2003): 614–36.

8. H. G. Koenig, H. Cohen, D. G. Blazer, et al., "Religious Coping and Depression in Elderly Hospitalized Medically Ill Men," *American Journal of Psychiatry* 149 (1992): 1693–1700.

9. H. G. Koenig, L. K. George, and B. L. Peterson, "Religiosity and Remission from Depression in Medically Ill Older Patients," *American Journal of Psychiatry* 155 (1998): 536–42.

10. H. G. Koenig, "Religion and Remission of Depression in Medical Inpatients with Heart Failure/Pulmonary Disease, *Journal of Nervous and Mental Disease* 195 (2007): 389–395.

11. J. B. Fenix, E. J. Cherlin, H. G. Prigerson, R. Johnson-Hurzeler, S. V. Kasl, and E. H. Bradley, "Religiousness and Major Depression among Bereaved Family Caregivers: A 13-Month Follow-Up Study," *Journal of Palliative Care* 22 (2006): 286–92.

12. Regarding a study examining anxiety, see J. Tauscher, R. M. Bagby, M. Javanmard, B. K. Christensen, S. Kasper, and S. Kapur, "Inverse Relationship between Serotonin 5-HT1A Receptor Binding and Anxiety: A [11C]WAY-100635 PET Investigation in Healthy Volunteers," *American Journal of Psychiatry* 158 (2001): 1326–28. For studies examining depression, see E. E. Bain, A. C. Nugent, R. E. Carson, et al., "Decreased 5-HT1A Receptor Binding in Bipolar Depression,"

*Biological Psychiatry* 55 (2004): Suppl.8;636; and P. A. Sargent, K. H. Kjaer, C. J. Bench, et al., "Brain Serotonin1a Receptor Binding Measured by Positron Emission Tomography with [11C]WAY-100635: Effects of Depression and Antidepressant Treatment," *Archives of General Psychiatry* 57 (2000): 174–80.

13. See the following: M. Z. Azhar and S. L. Varma, "Religious Psychotherapy in Depressive Patients," *Psychotherapy & Psychosomatics* 63 (1995): 165–73; L. R. Propst, "The Comparative Efficacy of Religious and Nonreligious Imagery for the Treatment of Mild Depression in Religious Individuals," *Cognitive Therapy & Research* 4 (1980): 167–78; L. R. Propst, R. Ostrom, P. Watkins, T. Dean, and D. Mashburn, "Comparative Efficacy of Religious and Nonreligious Cognitive-Behavior Therapy for the Treatment of Clinical Depression in Religious Individuals," *Journal of Consulting & Clinical Psychology* 60 (1992): 94–103; Y. M. Toh and S. Y. Tan, "The Effectiveness of Church-Based Lay Counselors: A Controlled Outcome Study," *Journal of Psychology & Christianity* 16 (1997): 260–67; and M. Z. Azhar and S. L. Varma, "Religious Psychotherapy as Management of Bereavement," *Acta Psychiatrica Scandinavica* 91 (1995): 233–35.

14. Koenig, McCullough, and Larson, *Handbook of Religion and Health*, 531–38.

15. F. Van Tubergen, M. Te Grotenhuis, and W. Ultee, "Denomination, Religious Context, and Suicide: Neo-Durkheimian Multilevel Explanations Tested with Individual and Contextual Data," *American Journal of Sociology* 111, no. 3 (2005): 797–823.

16. K. Dervic, M. A. Oquendo, M. F. Grunebaum, S. Ellis, A. K. Burke, and J. J. Mann, "Religious Affiliation and Suicide Attempt," *American Journal of Psychiatry* 161, no. 12 (2004): 2303–8.

17. L. Greening and L. Stoppelbein, "Religiosity, Attributional Style, and Social Support as Psychosocial Buffers for African American and White Adolescents' Perceived Risk for Suicide," *Suicide & Life-Threatening Behavior* 32, no. 4 (2002): 404–17.

18. C. S. McClain, B. Rosenfeld, and W. Breitbart, "Effect of Spiritual Well-Being on End-of-Life Despair in Terminally-Ill Cancer Patients," *Lancet* 361, no. 9369 (2003): 1603–7.

19. "Mental Health: A Report of the Surgeon General," 1999. See Web site: http://www.surgeongeneral.gov/library/mentalhealth/home.html

20. Koenig, McCullough, and Larson, *Handbook of Religion and Health*, 144–55, 536–38.

21. M. Speca, L. E. Carlson, E. Goodey, and M. Angen, "A Randomized, Wait-List Controlled Clinical Trial: The Effect of a Mindfulness Meditation-Based Stress Reduction Program on Mood and Symptoms of Stress in Cancer Outpatients," *Psychosomatic Medicine* 62, no. 5 (2000): 613–22.

22. P. Wink and J. Scott, "Does Religiousness Buffer against the Fear of Death and Dying in Late Adulthood? Findings from a Longitudinal Study," *Journal of Gerontology* 60, no. 4 (2005): P207–P214.

23. N. Boscaglia, D. M. Clarke, T. W. Jobling, and M. A. Quinn, "The Contribution of Spirituality and Spiritual Coping to Anxiety and Depression in Women with a Recent Diagnosis of Gynecological Cancer," *International Journal of Gynecological Cancer* 15, no. 5 (2005): 755–61.

24. K. I. Pargament, H. G. Koenig, N. Tarakeshwar, and J. Hahn, "Religious Cop-

ing Methods as Predictors of Psychological, Physical and Spiritual Outcomes among Medically Ill Elderly Patients: A Two-year Longitudinal Study," *Journal of Health Psychology* 9, no. 6 (2004): 713–30.

25. Koenig, McCullough, and Larson, *Handbook of Religion and Health*, 519–22.

26. J. M. Salsman, T. L. Brown, E. H. Brechting, and C. R. Carlson, "The Link between Religion and Spirituality and Psychological Adjustment: The Mediating Role of Optimism and Social Support," *Personality and Social Psychology Bulletin* 31, no. 4 (2005): 522–35.

27. N. Krause, "Religious Meaning and Subjective Well-Being in Late Life," *Journal of Gerontology* 58, no. 3 (2003): S160–70.

28. T. L. Krupski, L. Kwan, A. Fink, G. A. Sonn, S. Maliski, and M. S. Litwin, "Spirituality Influences Health Related Quality of Life in Men with Prostate Cancer," *Psycho-Oncology* 15, no. 2 (2006): 121–31.

29. E. Berman, J. F. Merz, M. Rudnick, et al., "Religiosity in a Hemodialysis Population and Its Relationship to Satisfaction with Medical Care, Satisfaction with Life, and Adherence," *American Journal of Kidney Diseases* 44, no. 3 (2004): 488–97.

30. Koenig, McCullough, and Larson, *Handbook of Religion and Health*, 522–23.

31. A. L. Ai, C. Peterson, T. N. Tice, S. F. Bolling, and H. G. Koenig, "Faith-based and Secular Pathways to Hope and Optimism Sub-Constructs in Middle-Aged and Older Cardiac Patients," *Journal of Health Psychology* 9, no. 3 (2004): 435–50.

32. S. Cotton, C. M. Puchalski, S. N. Sherman, et al., "Spirituality and Religion in Patients with HIV/AIDS," *Journal of General Internal Medicine* 21 (2006) (Suppl 5): S5–S13.

33. M. J. Pearce, J. L. Singer, and H. G. Prigerson, "Religious Coping among Caregivers of Terminally Ill Cancer Patients: Main Effects and Psychosocial Mediators," *Journal of Health Psychology* 11, no. 5 (2006): 743–59.

34. N. Krause, "Religious Meaning and Subjective Well-Being in Late Life," *Journal of Gerontology* 58, no. 3 (2003): S160–S170.

35. See C. McClain-Jacobson, B. Rosenfeld, A. Kosinski, H. Pessin, J. E. Cimino, and W. Breitbart, "Belief in an Afterlife, Spiritual Well-Being and End-of-Life Despair in Patients with Advanced Cancer," *General Hospital Psychiatry* 26, no. 6 (2004): 484–86; and C. S. McClain, B. Rosenfeld, and W. Breitbart, "Effect of Spiritual Well-Being on End-of-Life Despair in Terminally Ill Cancer Patients, " *Lancet* 361 (2003): 1603–7.

36. G. Ironson, G. F. Solomon, E. G. Balbin, et al., "Spirituality and Religiousness Are Associated with Long Survival, Health Behaviors, Less Distress, and Lower Cortisol in People Living with HIV/AIDS: The IWORSHIP Scale, Its Validity and Reliability," *Annals of Behavioral Medicine* 24 (2002): 34–48.

37. R. Arnold, S. K. Avants, A. Margolin, and D. Marcotte, "Patient Attitudes Concerning the Inclusion of Spirituality into Addiction Treatment," *Journal of Substance Abuse Treatment* 23, no. 4 (2002): 319–26.

38. S. Mohr, P. Y. Brandt, L. Borras, C. Gillieron, and P. Huguelet, "Toward an Integration of Spirituality and Religiousness into the Psychosocial Dimension of Schizophrenia," *American Journal of Psychiatry* 163, no. 11 (2006): 1952–59.

## CHAPTER 6: THE IMMUNE AND ENDOCRINE SYSTEMS

1. B. S. Rabin, *Stress, Immune Function, and Health: The Connection* (New York: Wiley-Liss & Sons, 1999).

2. D. C. McClelland, "The Effect of Motivational Arousal through Films on Salivary Immunoglobulin A," *Psychology and Health* 2 (1988): 31–52.

3. S. D. Harner, "Immune and Affect Response to Shamanic Drumming," *Dissertation Abstracts International* 56, no. 2-B (1995): 1108.

4. R. J. Davidson, J. Kabat-Zinn, J. Schumacher, et al., "Alterations in Brain and Immune Function Produced by Mindfulness Meditation," *Psychosomatic Medicine* 65, no. 4 (2003): 564–70.

5. T. E. Woods, M. H. Antoni, G. H. Ironson, and D. W. Kling, "Religiosity Is Associated with Affective and Immune Status in Symptomatic HIV-Infected Gay Men," *Journal of Psychosomatic Research* 46 (1999): 165–76.

6. S. E. Sephton, C. Koopman, M. Schaal, C. Thoreson, and D. Spiegel, "Spiritual Expression and Immune Status in Women with Metastatic Breast Cancer: An Exploratory Study," *Breast Journal* 7 (2001): 345–53.

7. G. Ironson, R. Stuetzie, and M. A. Flectcher, "An Increase in Religiousness/ Spirituality Occurs after HIV Diagnosis and Predicts Slower Disease Progression over 4 Years in People with HIV," *Journal of General Internal Medicine* 21 (2006): S62–S68.

8. Sephton, Koopman, Schaal, Thoreson, and Spiegel, "Spiritual Expression and Immune Status in Women with Metastatic Breast Cancer: An Exploratory Study."

9. H. Kimura, F. Nagao, Y. Tanaka, S. Sakai, S. Ohnishi, and K. Okumura, "Beneficial Effects of the Nishino Breathing Method on Immune Activity and Stress Level," *Journal of Alternative and Complementary Medicine* 11, no. 2 (2005): 285–91.

10. W. H. Koar, "Correlates of Meditation, Depression, Anxiety and T Cell Counts in HIV Positive Patients," *Dissertation Abstracts International* 56, no. 9-B (1996): 5174.

11. T. Kamei, Y. Toriumi, H. Kimura, and K. Kimura, "Correlation between Alpha Rhythms and Natural Killer Cell Activity during Yogic Respiratory Exercise," *Stress and Health: Journal of the International Society for the Investigation of Stress* 17, no. 3 (2001): 141–45.

12. H. G. Koenig, H. J. Cohen, L. K. George, J. C. Hays, D. B. Larson, and D. G. Blazer, "Attendance at Religious Services, Interleukin-6, and Other Biological Indicators of Immune Function in Older Adults," *International Journal of Psychiatry in Medicine* 27 (1997): 233–250. The Established Populations for Epidemiologic Studies in the Elderly (EPESE) is a longitudinal study supported by the National Institute on Aging, part of the National Institutes of Health. A random sample of over 14,000 persons aged sixty-five or older was originally selected in the 1980s from four sites: East Boston, New Haven, Iowa, and central North Carolina. Follow-up has occurred every 1.5-to-3 years of this cohort through the mid-1990s. In 1993–94, the Hispanic EPESE was conducted in southern Texas, surveying an additional 3,050 older Mexican Americans, who have been followed up yearly through 2006. The central North Carolina site of the EPESE included 4,000 older adults and was run by investigators at

Duke University Medical Center. The purpose of the EPESE was to examine psychological, social, demographic, and other characteristics of community-dwelling older adults that might influence their health and well-being as they aged.

13. S. K. Lutgendorf, D. Russell, P. Ullrich, T. B. Harris, and R. Wallace, "Religious Participation, Interleukin-6, and Mortality in Older Adults," *Health Psychology* 23, no. 5 (2004): 465–75.

14. C. M. Jacobson, "Exploring the Mind-Body Connection: Spirituality, Religiosity, and Immune Functioning in Patients with Terminal Cancer," *Dissertation Abstracts International 66*, no. 3-B. (2005): 1720.

15. D. M. Yeager, D. A. Glei, M.Au, H. S. Lin, R. P. Sloan, and M. Weinstein, "Religious Involvement and Health Outcomes among Older Persons in Taiwan," *Social Sciences and Medicine 63* no. 8 (2006): 2228–41.

16. J. K. Neumann and D. S. Chi "Relationship of Church Giving to Immunological and TxPA Stress Response," *Journal of Psychology & Theology* 27, no. 1 (1999): 43–51.

17. L. E. Carlson, M. Speca, K. D. Patel, and E. Goodey, "Mindfulness-based Stress Reduction in Relation to Quality of Life, Mood, Symptoms of Stress, and Immune Parameters in Breast and Prostate Cancer Outpatients," *Psychosomatic Medicine* 65, no. 4 (2003): 571–81.

18. H. G. Koenig, M. E. McCullough, and D. B. Larson, *Handbook of Religion and Health* (New York: Oxford University Press, 2001), 560.

19. J. Katz, H. Weiner, T. Gallagher, et al., "Stress, Distress, and Ego Defenses," *Archives of General Psychiatry* 23 (1970): 131–42.

20. M. D. Schaal, S. E. Sephton, C. Thoreson, C. Koopman, and D. Spiegel, "Religious Expression and Immune Competence in Women with Advanced Cancer," paper presented at the Annual Meeting of the American Psychological Association, San Francisco, CA, August 1998. See also notes 6 and 8 in this chapter.

21. G. Ironson, G. F. Solomon, E. G. Balbin, et al., "Spirituality and Religiousness Are Associated with Long Survival, Health Behaviors, Less Distress, and Lower Cortisol in People Living with HIV/AIDS: The IWORSHIP Scale, Its Validity and Reliability," *Annals of Behavioral Medicine* 24 (2002): 34–48.

22. E. A. Dedert, J. L. Studts, I. Weissbecker, P. G. Salmon, P. L. Banis, and S. E. Sephton, "Private Religious Practice: Protection of Cortisol Rhythms among Women with Fibromyalgia," *International Journal of Psychiatry in Medicine* 34 (2004): 61–77.

23. J. Tartaro, L. J. Luecken, and H. E. Gunn, "Exploring Heart and Soul: Effects of Religiosity/Spirituality and Gender on Blood Pressure and Cortisol Stress Responses," *Journal of Health Psychology* 10, no. 6 (2005): 753–66.

24. M. S. Lee, M. K. Kim, and H. Ryu, "Qi-Training (Qigong) Enhanced Immune Functions: What Is the Underlying Mechanism?" *International Journal of Neuroscience* 115, no. 8 (2005): 1099–1104.

25. C. P. Donahue, K. S. Kosik, and T. J. Shors, "Growth Hormone Is Produced within the Hippocampus Where It Responds to Age, Sex, and Stress," *Proceedings of the National Academy of Sciences of the United States of America* 103, no. 15 (2006): 6031–36.

26. M. S. Lee, H. Ryu, and H. T. Chung, "Stress Management by Psychosomatic

Training: Effects of Cundosunbup Qi-Training on Symptoms of Stress—Cross-Sectional Study," *Stress Medicine* 16, no. 3 (2000): 161–66.
27. Yeager, Glei, Au, Lin, Sloan, and Weinstein, "Religious Involvement and Health . . . in Taiwan."

## Chapter 7: The Cardiovascular System

1. H. G. Koenig, M. E. McCullough, and D. B. Larson, *Handbook of Religion and Health* (New York: Oxford University Press 2001), 557–58.

2. H. G. Koenig, L. K. George, H. J. Cohen, et al., "The Relationship between Religious Activities and Blood Pressure in Older Adults," *International Journal of Psychiatry in Medicine* 28 (1998): 189–213.

3. M. Timio, P. Verdecchia, S. Venanzi, et al., "Age and Blood Pressure Changes: A 20-Year Follow-Up Study in Nuns in a Secluded Order," *Hypertension* 12 (1988): 457–61.

4. K. Newlin, G. D. Melkus, D. Chyun, and V. Jefferson, "The Relationship of Spirituality and Health Outcomes in Black Women with Type II Diabetes," *Ethnicity & Disease* 13, no. 1 (2003): 61–68.

5. J. van Olphen, A. Schulz, B. Israel, et al., "Religious Involvement, Social Support, and Health among African-American Women on the East Side of Detroit," *Journal of General Internal Medicine* 18, no. 7 (2003): 549–57.

6. P. R. Steffen and A. L. Hinderliter, "Religious Coping, Ethnicity, and Ambulatory Blood Pressure," *Psychosomatic Medicine* 63, no. 4 (2001): 523–30.

7. R. F. Gillum and D. D. Ingram, "Frequency of Attendance at Religious Services, Hypertension, and Blood Pressure: The Third National Health and Nutrition Examination Survey," *Psychosomatic Medicine* 68 (2006): 382–85.

8. G. Rose, "Strategy of Prevention: Lessons from Cardiovascular Disease," *Board Medical Journal* 282 (1981): 1847–55.

9. M. G. Marmot, "Diet, Hypertension, and Stroke," in *Nutrition and Health*, ed. M. R. Turner (New York: Alan R. Liss Publishers, 1982), 243.

10. N. Krause, J. Liang J, et al., "Religion, Death of a Loved One, and Hypertension among Older Adults in Japan," *Journals of Gerontology Series B: Psychological Sciences and Social Sciences* 57B, no. 2 (2002): S96–S107.

11. D. M. Yeager, D. A. Glei, M. Au, H. S. Lin, R. P. Sloan, and M. Weinstein, "Religious Involvement and Health Outcomes among Older Persons in Taiwan," *Social Sciences and Medicine* 63, no. 8 (2006): 2228–41.

12. Y. Y. Al-Kandari, "Religiosity and Its Relation to Blood Pressure among Selected Kuwaitis," *Journal of Biosocial Science* 35 (2003): 463–72.

13. F. A. Treiber, T. Kamarck, N. Schneiderman et al., "Cardiovascular Reactivity and Development of Preclinical and Clinical Disease States," *Psychosomatic Medicine* 65 (2003): 46–62.

14. Y. Y. Chen, S. Gilligan, E. Coups, and R. J. Contrada, "Religiousness and Cardiovascular Reactivity, paper read at the 109th Annual Convention of the American Psychological Association. San Francisco, CA, August 2001.

15. J. Tartaro, L. J. Luecken, and H. E. Gunn, "Exploring Heart and Soul: Effects of Religiosity/Spirituality and Gender on Blood Pressure and Cortisol Stress Responses," *Journal of Health Psychology* 10, no. 6 (2005): 753–66.

16. K. S. Masters, R. D. Hill, J. C. Kircher, T. L. Benson, and J. A. Fallon, "Religious Orientation, Aging, and Blood Pressure Reactivity to Interpersonal and Cognitive Stressors," *Annals of Behavioral Medicine* 28, no. 3 (2004): 171–78.

17. Koenig, McCullough, and Larson, *Handbook of Religion and Health,* 557–58.

18. R. H. Schneider, F. Staggers, C. Alexander, et al., "A Randomized Controlled Trial of Stress Reduction for Hypertension in Older African Americans," *Hypertension* 26 (1995): 820–29.

19. S. R. Wenneberg, R. H. Schneider, K. G. Walton, et al., "A Controlled Study for the Effects of the Transcendental Meditation Program on Cardiovascular Reactivity and Ambulatory Blood Pressure," *International Journal of Neuroscience* 89, nos. 1–2 (1997), 15–28.

20. R. H. Schneider, C. N. Alexander, F. Staggers, et al., "A Randomized Controlled Trial of Stress Reduction in African Americans Treated for Hypertension for over One Year," *American Journal of Hypertension* 18, no. 1 (2005): 88–98.

21. K. Harinath, A. S. Malhotra, K. Pal, et al., "Effects of Hatha Yoga and Omkar Meditation on Cardiorespiratory Performance, Psychologic Profile, and Melatonin Secretion," *Journal of Alternative and Complementary Medicine* 10 (2004): 261–68.

22. M. Paul-Labrador, D. Polk, J. H. Dwyer, et al., "Effects of a Randomized Controlled Trial of Transcendental Meditation on Components of the Metabolic Syndrome in Subjects with Coronary Heart Disease," *Archives of Internal Medicine* 166, no. 11 (2006): 1218–24.

23. A. Castillo-Richmond, R. H. Schneider, C. N. Alexander, et al., "Effects of Stress Reduction on Carotid Atherosclerosis in Hypertensive African Americans," *Stroke* 31, no. 3 (2000): 568–73.

24. L. Bernardi, P. Sleight, G. Bandinelli, et al., "Effect of Rosary Prayer and Yoga Mantras on Autonomic Cardiovascular Rhythms: Comparative Study," *British Medical Journal* 323, no. 7327 (2001): 1446–49.

25. M. T. La Rovere, J. T. Bigger Jr, F. I. Marcus, A. Mortara, and P. J. Schwartz, "Baroreflex Sensitivity and HeartRate Variability in Prediction of Total Cardiac Mortality after Myocardial Infarction," *Lancet* 351 (1998): 478–84.

26. P. Ernsberger and D. O. Nelson, "Effects of Fasting and Refeeding on Blood Pressure Are Determined by Nutritional State, Not by Body Weight Change," *American Journal of Hypertension* 1 (1988): 153S–157S.

27. G. Perk, J. Ghanem, S. Aamar, D. Ben-Ishay, and M. Bursztyn, "The Effect of the Fast of Ramadan on Ambulatory Blood Pressure in Treated Hypertensives," *Journal of Human Hypertension* 15, no. 10 (2001): 723–25.

28. G. E. Frazer, T. M. Strahan, J. Sabate, W. L. Beeson, and D. Kissinger, "Effects of Traditional Coronary Risk Factors on Rates of Incident Coronary Events in a Low-Risk Population: The Adventist Health Study," *Circulation* 86 (1992): 406–13.

29. A. Adlouni, et al., "Fasting during Ramadan Induces a Marked Increase in High-Density Lipoprotein Cholesterol and Decrease in Low-Density Lipoprotein Cholesterol," *Annals of Nutrition and Metabolism* 41 (1997): 242–49.

30. Y. Friedlander, J. D. Kark, and Y. Stein, "Religious Observance and Plasma Lipids and Lipoproteins among 17-Year-Old Jewish Residents of Jerusalem," *Preventive Medicine* 16 (1987): 70–79.

31. Koenig, McCullough, and Larson, *Handbook of Religion and Health*, 569.

32. W. J. Strawbridge, R. D. Cohen, S. J. Shema, and G. A. Kaplan, "Frequent Attendance at Religious Services and Mortality over 28 Years," *American Journal of Public Health* 87 (1997): 957–61. The Alameda County Study is a major epidemiological study that involved a sample of nearly 7,000 randomly selected persons in Alameda County, just east of the San Francisco Bay Area in California. Participants, ages seventeen to ninety-four, were first surveyed in the mid-1960s and followed for nearly thirty years through 1994. An original focus of the study was to evaluate the effects of social factors (social support, social activity, social memberships) on mental and physical health. Literally hundreds of papers have been published using data from the Alameda County Study that have demonstrated the impact of social activities on health and longevity.

33. D. McIntosh and B. Spilka, "Religion and Physical Health: The Role of Personal Faith and Control Beliefs," *Research in the Social Scientific Study of Religion* 2 (1990): 167–94.

34. K. H. Kim and J. Sobal, "Religion, Social Support, Fat Intake and Physical Activity," *Public Health Nutrition* 7, no. 6 (2004): 773–81.

35. R. M. Merrill and A. L. Thygerson, "Religious Preference, Church Activity, and Physical Exercise," *Preventive Medicine* 33, no. 1 (2001): 38–45.

36. D. R. Young and K. J. Stewart, "A Church-Based Physical Activity Intervention for African American Women," *Family & Community Health* 29, no. 2 (2006): 103–17.

37. Koenig, McCullough, and Larson, *Handbook of Religion and Health*, 570–71.

38. H. G. Koenig, L. K. George, H. J. Cohen, J. C. Hays, D. G. Blazer, and D. B. Larson, "The Relationship between Religious Activities and Cigarette Smoking in Older Adults," *Journals of Gerontology Series A: Biological Sciences and Medical Sciences* 53A (1998): M426–M434.

## Chapter 8: Diseases Related to Stress and Behavior

1. G. W. Comstock, "Fatal Arteriosclerotic Heart Disease, Water Hardness at Home, and Socioeconomic Characteristics," *American Journal of Epidemiology* 94 (1971): 1–10.

2. H. G. Koenig, "Editorial: Religion, Spirituality and Medicine: How Are They Related and What Does It Mean?" *Mayo Clinic Proceedings* 76 (2001): 1189–91. See also, H. G. Koenig, "Health-prayer studies." *Science & Spirit Magazine*, March–April (2002): 20-22 (see http://www.science-spirit.org/article_detail.php?article_id=295; last accessed 12/28/07).

3. Y. Friedlander, J. D. Kark, and Y. Stein, "Religious Orthodoxy and Myocardial Infarction in Jerusalem—A Case-Control Study," *International Journal of Cardiology* 10 (1986): 33–41.

4. U. Goldbourt, S. Yaari, and J. H. Medalie, "Factors Predictive of Long-Term Coronary Heart Disease Mortality among 10,059 Male Israeli Civil Servants and Municipal Employees," *Cardiology* 82 (1993): 100–21.

5. R. Gupta, H. Prakash, V. P. Gupta, and K. D. Gupta, "Prevalence and Determinants of Coronary Heart Disease in a Rural Population of India, *Journal of Clinical Epidemiology* 50 (1997): 203–9.

6. N. Gopinath, S. L. Chadha, P. Jain, S. Shekhawat, and R. Tandon, "An Epidemiological Study of Coronary Heart Disease in Different Ethnic Groups in Delhi Urban Population," *Journal of the Association of Physicians of India* 43, no. 1 (1995): 30–33.

7. R. L. Phillips, J. W. Kuzma, W. L. Beeson, and T. Lotz, "Influence of Selection versus Lifestyle on Risk of Fatal Cancer and Cardiovascular Disease among Seventh-day Adventists," *American Journal of Epidemiology* 112 (1980): 296–314.

8. J. W. Zamarra, R. H. Schneider, I. Besseghini, D. K. Robinson, and J. W. Salerno, "Usefulness of the Transcendental Meditation Program in the Treatment of Patients with Coronary Artery Disease," *American Journal of Cardiology* 77 (1996): 867–70.

9. P. Yelsma, and L. Montambo, "Patients' and Spouses' Religious Problem-Solving Styles and Their Physiological Health," *Psychological Reports* 66 (1990): 857–58.

10. M. Agrawal, Manju, and A.K. Dalal. "Beliefs about the World and Recovery from Myocardial Infarction, *Journal of Social Psychology* 133(1993):385-394.

11. T. E. Oxman, D. H. Freeman, and E. D. Manheimer, "Lack of Social Participation or Religious Strength and Comfort as Risk Factors for Death after Cardiac Surgery in the Elderly," *Psychosomatic Medicine* 57 (1995): 5–15.

12. R. J. Contrada, T. M. Goyal, C. Cather, L. Rafalson, E. L. Idler, and T. J. Krause, "Psychosocial Factors in Outcomes of Heart Surgery: The Impact of Religious Involvement and Depressive Symptoms," *Health Psychology* 23 (2004): 227–38.

13. A. L. Ai, C. Peterson, S. F. Bolling, and W. Rodgers, "Depression, Faith-based Coping, and Short-term Postoperative Global Functioning in Adult and Older Patients Undergoing Cardiac Surgery," *Journal of Psychosomatic Research* 60, no. 1 (2006): 21–28.

14. A. Castillo-Richmond, R. H. Schneider, C. N. Alexander, et al., "Effects of Stress Reduction on Carotid Atherosclerosis in Hypertensive African Americans," *Stroke* 31, no. 3 (2000): 568–73.

15. Regarding research on Mormons, see G. K. Jarvis, "Mormon Mortality Rates in Canada," *Social Biology* 24 (1977): 294–302. Regarding a study on Seventh-day Adventists, see Phillips, Kuzma, Beeson, and Lotz, "Influence of Selection versus Lifestyle on Risk of Fatal Cancer and Cardiovascular Disease among Seventh-day Adventists.

16. A. Colantonio, S. V. Kasl, and A. M. Ostfeld, "Depressive Symptoms and Other Psychosocial Factors as Predictors of Stroke in Elderly," *American Journal of Epidemiology* 136 (1992): 884–94.

17. M. R. Benjamins, M. A. Musick, D. T. Gold, and L. K.George, "Age-related Declines in Activity Level: The Relationship between Chronic Illness and Religious Activities," *Journals of Gerontology Series B: Psychological Sciences and Social Sciences* 58, no. 6 (2003): S377–S385.

18. P. H. Van Ness, and S. V. Kasl, "Religion and Cognitive Dysfunction in an Elderly Cohort," *Journal of Gerontology* 58B, no. 1 (2003): S21–S29.

19. Y. Kaufman and M. Freedman, "Religion, Spirituality May Slow Alzheimer's," paper presented at the 57th Meeting of the American Academy of Neurology, Miami Beach, Florida, April 9–16, 2005; later published as Y. Kaufman,

D. Anaki, M. Binns, and M. Freedman, "Cognitive Decline in Alzheimer's Disease: Impact of Spirituality, Religiosity, and QOL," *Neurology* 68 (2007): 1509–14.

20. R. D. Hill, A. M. Burdette, J. L. Angel, and R. J. Angel, "Religious Attendance and Cognitive Functioning among Older Mexican Americans," *Journals of Gerontology Series B: Psychological Sciences and Social Sciences* 61, no. 1 (2006): P3–P9.

21. D. M. Yeager, D. A. Glei, M. Au, H. S. Lin, R. P. Sloan, and M. Weinstein, "Religious Involvement and Health Outcomes among Older Persons in Taiwan," *Social Sciences and Medicine* 63, no. 8 (2006): 2228–41.

22. M. R. Carnethon, M. L. Biggs, J. I. Barzilay, et al., "Longitudinal Association between Depressive Symptoms and Incident Type II Diabetes Mellitus in Older Adults," *Archives of Internal Medicine* 167 (2007): 802–7.

23. J. van Olphen, A. Schulz, B. Israel, et al., "Religious Involvement, Social Support, and Health among African-American Women on the East Side of Detroit," *Journal of General Internal Medicine* 18, no. 7 (2003): 549–57.

24. K. Newlin, "The Relationship of Religion and Spirituality to Blood Glucose Control in Black Women with Type II Diabetes" (PhD diss., Yale University, New Haven, CT, 2007).

25. D. E. King, A. G. Mainous III, and W. S. Pearson, "C-reactive Protein, Diabetes, and Attendance at Religious Services," *Diabetes Care* 25, no. 7 (2002): 1172–76.

26. K. Newlin, G. D. Melkus, D. Chyun, and V. Jefferson, "The Relationship of Spirituality and Health Outcomes in Black Women with Type II Diabetes," *Ethnicity & Disease* 13, no. 1 (2003): 61–68.

27. A. G. Naeem, "The Role of Culture and Religion in the Management of Diabetes: A Study of Kashmiri Men in Leeds," *Journal of the Royal Society of Health* 123, no. 2 (2003): 110–16.

28. See, for example, C. S. McClain, B. Rosenfeld, and W. Breitbart, "Effect of Spiritual Well-being on End-of-Life Despair in Terminally-ill Cancer Patients," *Lancet* 361, no. 9369 (2003): 1603–7; and E. S. Samano, P. T. Goldenstein, M. Ribeiro Lde, et al., "Praying Correlates with Higher Quality of Life: Results from a Survey on Complementary/Alternative Medicine Use among a Group of Brazilian Cancer Patients," *Sao Paulo Medical Journal* 122, no. 2 (2004): 60–63.

29. For studies on Seventh-day Adventists, see F. R. Lemon and R. T. Walden, "Death from Respiratory System Disease among Seventh-day Adventist Men," *Journal of the American Medical Association* 198 (1966): 137–46; J. Berkel and F. de Waard, "Mortality Pattern and Life Expectancy of Seventh-day Adventists in The Netherlands," *International Journal of Epidemiology* 12 (1983): 455–59; and G. E. Fraser, W. L. Beeson, and R. L. Phillips, "Diet and Lung Cancer in California Seventh-day Adventists," *American Journal of Epidemiology* 133 (1991): 683–93. For studies on Mormons, see J. L. Lyon, M. R. Klauber, J. W. Gardner, and C. R. Smart, "Cancer Incidence in Mormons and Non-Mormons in Utah, 1966–1970," *New England Journal of Medicine* 294 (1976): 129–33; and J. E. Enstrom, "Health Practices and Cancer Mortality among Active California Mormons," *Journal of the National Cancer Institute* 31 (1989): 1807–14. For a study on the Amish, see R. F. Hamman, J. I. Barancik, and A. M. Lilienfeld, "Patterns of Mortality in the Old Order Amish," *American Journal of Epidemiology* 114 (1981): 845–61. Finally,

for a study on other religions with prohibitions against negative health behaviors, see A. O. Martin, J. K. Dunn, J. L. Simpson, et al., "Cancer Mortality in a Human Isolate," *Journal of the National Cancer Institute* 65 (1980): 1109–13.

30. Enstrom, "Health Practices and Cancer Mortality among Active California Mormons."

31. G. Ringdal, K. Gotestam, S. Kaasa, S. Kvinnslaud, and K. Ringdal, (1995). Prognostic Factors and Survival in a Heterogeneous Sample of Cancer Patients. *British Journal of Cancer* 73, (1995) 1594–99; also see, G. Ringdal "Religiosity, Quality of Life and Survival in Cancer Patients." *Social Indicators Research* 38, 193–211.

32. D. Oman, J. H. Kurata, W. J. Strawbridge, and R. D. Cohen, "Religious Attendance and Cause of Death over 31 Years," *International Journal of Psychiatry in Medicine* 32, no. 1 (2002): 69–89.

33. G. A. Kune, S. Kune, and L. F. Watson, "Perceived Religiousness Is Protective for Colorectal Cancer: Data from the Melbourne Colorectal Cancer Study," *Journal of the Royal Society of Medicine* 86, no. 11 (1993): 645–47.

34. R. Hummer, R. Rogers, C. Nam, and C. G. Ellison, "Religious Involvement and U.S. Adult Mortality," *Demography* 36 (1999): 273–85.

35. L. H. Powell, L. Shahabi, and C. E. Thoresen, "Religion and Spirituality: Linkages to Physical Health," *American Psychologist* 58 (2003): 36–52.

36. See G. E. Wilson, "Christian Science and Longevity," *Journal of Forensic Science* 1 (1965): 43–60; W. F. Simpson, "Comparative Longevity in a College Cohort of Christian Scientists," *Journal of the American Medical Association* 262 (1989): 1657–58; and J. Mitchell, D. R. Lannin, H. F. Mathews, and M. S. Swanson, "Religious Beliefs and Breast Cancer Screening," *Journal of Women's Health* 11 (2002): 907–15.

## CHAPTER 9: LONGEVITY

1. J. v. B. Hjelmborg, I. Iachine, A. Skytthe, et al., "Genetic Influence on Human Lifespan and Longevity," *Human Genetics* 119, no. 3 (2006): 312–21.

2. A. Macieira-Coelho, *Biology of Aging* (New York: Springer, 2002), 48.

3. G. Kolata, "Live Long? Die Young? Answer Isn't Just in Genes," *New York Times*, August 31, 2006. See http://www.nytimes.com/2006/08/31/health/31age.html?ex=1177732800&en=3735f45810a0a9e1&ei=5070 (last accessed 4/30/07).

4. Regarding causes of death in the United States, see A. H. Mokdad, J. S. Marks, D. F. Stroup, and J. L. Gerberding, "Actual Causes of Death in the United States, 2000," *Journal of the American Medical Association* 291 (2004): 1238–45. Concerning worldwide causes of death, see "World Health Report 1999 database. Table 1. Leading Causes of Death, Both Sexes, 1998." See http://whqlibdoc.who.int/hq/1999/WHO_HSC_PVI_99.11.pdf (last accessed 4/30/07).

5. R. P. Sloan, *Blind Faith: The Unholy Alliance between Religion and Medicine* (New York: St. Martin's Press, 2006), 143–47.

6. See the following studies: W. J. Strawbridge, R. D. Cohen, S. J. Shema, and G. A. Kaplan, "Frequent Attendance at Religious Services and Mortality over 28 Years," *American Journal of Public Health* 87 (1997): 957–61; W. J. Strawbridge, S. J. Shema, R. D. Cohen, and G. A. Kaplan, "Religious Attendance Increases

Survival by Improving and Maintaining Good Health Behaviors, Mental Health, and Social Relationships," *Annals of Behavioral Medicine* 23 (2001): 68–74; H. G. Koenig, L. K. George, and B. L. Peterson, "Religiosity and Remission from Depression in Medically Ill Older Patients," *American Journal of Psychiatry* 155 (1998): 536–42; and H. G. Koenig, "Religion and Remission of Depression in Medical Inpatients with Heart Failure/Pulmonary Disease," *Journal of Nervous and Mental Disease* 195 (2007): 389–95.

7. A. B. Hill, "The Environment and Disease: Association or Causation?" *Proceedings of the Royal Society of Medicine* 58 (1965): 295–300 (Hill's criteria for causation).

8. M. E. McCullough, W. T. Hoyt, D. B. Larson, H. G. Koenig, and C. Thoresen, "Religious Involvement and Mortality: A Meta-Analytic Review," *Health Psychology* 19, no. 3 (2000): 211–22.

9. See the following: Strawbridge, Cohen, Shema, and Kaplan, "Frequent Attendance at Religious Services and Mortality Over 28 Years"; R. A. Hummer, R. G. Rogers, C. B. Nam, and C. G. Ellison, "Religious Involvement and U.S. Adult Mortality," *Demography* 36 (1999): 273–85; H. G. Koenig, J. C. Hays, D. B. Larson, et al., "Does Religious Attendance Prolong Survival?: A Six-Year Follow-Up Study of 3,968 Older Adults," *Journal of Gerontology Series A, Biological Sciences and Medical Sciences* 54A (1999): M370–M376; M. A. Musick, J. S. House, and D. R. Williams, "Attendance at Religious Services and Mortality in a National Sample," *Journal of Health and Social Behavior* 45 (2004): 198–213.

10. L. H. Powell, L. Shahabi, and C. E. Thoresen, "Religion and Spirituality: Linkages to Physical Health," *American Psychologist* 58, no. 1 (2003): 36–52.

11. M. E. McCullough, "Religious Involvement and Mortality: Answers and More Questions," in *Faith and Health*, eds. T. G. Plante and A. C. Sherman, 53–74 (New York: Guilford, 2001).

12. See J. A. Jolliffe, K. Rees, R. S. Taylor, D. Thompson, N. Oldridge, and S. Ebrahim, "Exercise-Based Rehabilitation for Coronary Heart Disease" [computer file], *The Cochrane Database of Systematic Reviews* 4 (2000), CD001800. Cochrane Collaboration

13. G. D. Smith, F. Song, and T. A. Sheldon, "Cholesterol Lowering and Mortality: The Importance of Considering Initial Level of Risk," *British Medical Journal* 306 (1993): 1367–73.

14. W. Linden, C. Stossel, and J. Maurice, "Psychosocial Interventions for Patients with Coronary Artery Disease: A Meta-Analysis," *Archives of Internal Medicine* 156 (1996): 745–52.

15. C. D. Holman, D. R. English, E. Milne, and M. G. Winter, "Meta-Analysis of Alcohol and All-Cause Mortality: A Validation of the NHMRC Recommendations," *Medical Journal of Australia* 164 (1996): 141–45.

16. D. E. Hall, "Religious Attendance: More Cost-Effective Than Lipitor?" *Journal of the American Board of Family Medicine* 19 (2006): 103–9.

17. Strawbridge, Cohen, Shema, and Kaplan, "Frequent Attendance at Religious Services and Mortality over 28 Years."

18. W. J. Strawbridge, R. D. Cohen, and S. J. Shema, "Comparative Strength of Association between Religious Attendance and Survival," *International Journal of Psychiatry in Medicine* 30, no. 4 (2000): 299–308.

19. Strawbridge, Shema, Cohen, and Kaplan, "Religious Attendance Increases Survival by Improving and Maintaining Good Health Behaviors, Mental Health, and Social Relationships."

20. Hummer, Rogers, Nam, and Ellison, "Religious Involvement and U.S. Adult Mortality."

21. H. G. Koenig, J. C. Hays, D. B. Larson et al., "Does Religious Attendance Prolong Survival?: M370–M376.

22. P. la Cour, K. Avlund, and K. Schultz-Larsen, "Religion and Survival in a Secular Region: A Twenty Year Follow-up of 734 Danish Adults Born in 1914." *Social Science & Medicine* 62 (2006): 157–164.

23. D. M. Yeager, D. A. Glei, M. Au, H. S. Lin, R. P. Sloan, and M. Weinstein, "Religious Involvement and Health Outcomes among Older Persons in Taiwan," *Social Sciences and Medicine* 63, no. 8 (2006): 2228–41.

24. See the following studies: K. I. Pargament, H. G. Koenig, N. Tarakeshwar, and J. Hahn, "Religious Struggle as a Predictor of Mortality among Medically Ill Elderly Patients: A Two-Year Longitudinal Study," *Archives of Internal Medicine* 161 (2001): 1881–85; C. N. Alexander, E. J. Langer, R. I. Newman, H. M. Chandler, and J. L. Davies, "Transcendental Meditation, Mindfulness, and Longevity: An Experimental Study with the Elderly," *Journal of Personality and Social Psychology* 57 (1989): 950–64; H. M. Helm, J. C. Hays, E. P. Flint, H. G. Koenig, and D. G. Blazer. "Does Private Religious Activity Prolong Survival? A Six-Year Follow-Up Study of 3,851 Older Adults," *Journals of Gerontology Series A: Biological Sciences and Medical Sciences* 55 (2000): M400–M405; and Yeager, Glei, Au, Lin, Sloan, and Weinstein, "Religious Involvement and Health Outcomes among Older Persons in Taiwan."

25. Alexander, Langer, Newman, Chandler, and Davies, "Transcendental Meditation, Mindfulness, and Longevity: An Experimental Study with the Elderly."

26. Yeager, Glei, Au, Lin, Sloan, and Weinstein, "Religious Involvement and Health Outcomes among Older Persons in Taiwan."

27. Helm, Hays, Flint, Koenig, and Blazer, "Does Private Religious Activity Prolong Survival? A Six-Year Follow-Up Study of 3,851 Older Adults."

28. A. L.Ai, C. Peterson, S. F. Bolling, and W. Rodgers, "Depression, Faith-Based Coping, and Short-Term Postoperative Global Functioning in Adult and Older Patients Undergoing Cardiac Surgery," *Journal of Psychosomatic Research* 60 (2006): 21–28.

29. R. J. Contrada, T. M. Goyal, C. Cather, L. Rafalson, E. L. Idler, and T. J. Krause, "Psychosocial Factors in Outcomes of Heart Surgery: The Impact of Religious Involvement and Depressive Symptoms," *Health Psychology* 23 (2004): 227–38.

30. D. A. Matthews, S. M. Marlowe, et al., "Effects of Intercessory Prayer on Patients with Rheumatoid Arthritis," *Southern Medical Journal* 93 (2000): 1177–86.

31. Pargament, Koenig, Tarakeshwar, and Hahn, "Religious Struggle as a Predictor of Mortality among Medically Ill Elderly Patients: A Two-Year Longitudinal Study."

CHAPTER 10: PHYSICAL DISABILITY

1. See R. J. Turner and S. Noh, "Physical Disability and Depression: A Longitudinal Analysis," *Journal of Health & Social Behavior* 29, no. 1 (1988): 23–37; and H.

G. Koenig, J. L. Johnson, and B. L. Peterson, "Major Depression and Physical Illness Trajectories in Heart Failure and Pulmonary Disease," *Journal of Nervous and Mental Disease* 194 (2006): 909–16.

2. J. T. Newsom and R. Schulz, "Caregiving from the Recipient's Perspective: Negative Reactions to Being Helped," *Health Psychology* 17 (1998): 172–81.

3. See the following studies: S. Rinaldi, M. Ghisi, L. Iaccarino, et al., "Influence of Coping Skills on Health-Related Quality of Life in Patients with Systemic Lupus Erythematosus," *Arthritis & Rheumatism* 55, no. 3 (2006): 427–33; M. G. Njoku, L. A. Jason, and S. R. Torres-Harding, "The Relationships among Coping Styles and Fatigue in an Ethnically Diverse Sample," *Ethnicity & Health* 10, no. 4 (2005): 263–78; A. L. Stanton, S. Danoff-Burg, and M. E. Huggins, "The First Year after Breast Cancer Diagnosis: Hope and Coping Strategies as Predictors of Adjustment," *Psycho-Oncology* 11, no. 2 (2002): 93–102; and C. Zwingmann, M. Wirtz, C. Muller, J. Korber, and S. Murken, "Positive and Negative Religious Coping in German Breast Cancer Patients," *Journal of Behavioral Medicine* 29, no. 6 (2006): 533–47.

4. C. J. L. Murray and A. D. Lopez, *The Global Burden of Disease* (Cambridge, MA: Harvard University Press, 1996), cited in *British Medical Journal* 325 (2002): 947.

5. See R. F. Guy, "Religion, Physical Disabilities, and Life Satisfaction in Older Age Cohorts," *International Journal of Aging & Human Development* 15, no. 3 (1982): 225–32; and H. G. Koenig, J. N. Kvale, and C. Ferrel, "Religion and Well-being in Later Life," *The Gerontologist* 28 (1988): 18–28.

6. H. G. Koenig, H. J. Cohen, D. G. Blazer, et al., "Religious Coping and Depression in Elderly Hospitalized Medically Ill Men," *American Journal of Psychiatry* 149 (1992): 1693–1700.

7. H. G. Koenig, L. K. George, and B. L. Peterson, "Religiosity and Remission from Depression in Medically Ill Older Patients," *American Journal of Psychiatry* 155 (1998): 536–42.

8. P. Pressman, J. S. Lyons, D. B. Larson, and J. J. Strain, "Religious Belief, Depression, and Ambulation Status in Elderly Women with Broken Hips," *American Journal of Psychiatry* 147 (1990): 758–59.

9. E. L. Idler and S. V. Kasl, "Religion among Disabled and Nondisabled Elderly Persons, II: Attendance at Religious Services as a Predictor of the Course of Disability," *Journal of Gerontology* 52B (1997): S306–S316.

10. R. M. Allman, P. Sawyer-Baker, R. M. Maisiak, R. V. Sims, and J. M. Roseman, "Racial Similarities and Differences in Predictors of Mobility Change over Eighteen Months," *Journal of Geriatric Internal Medicine* 19 (2004): 1118–26.

11. R. J. Taylor, "Religious Participation among Elderly Blacks," *Gerontologist* 26 (1986): 630–36.

12. M. R. Benjamins, "Religion and Functional Health among the Elderly: Is There a Relationship and Is It Constant?" *Journal of Aging and Health* 16 (2004): 355–74.

13. N. S. Park, D. L. Klemmack, L. L. Roff, M. W. Parker, H. G. Koenig, P. Sawyer, and R. L. Allman, "Religiousness and Longitudinal Trajectories in Elders' Functional Status," *Research on Aging*, in press (2008).

14. J. A. Kelley-Moore and K. F. Ferraro, "Functional Limitations and Religious

Service Attendance in Later Life: Barrier and/or Benefit Mechanism?" *Journal of Gerontology Saries B: Psychological Sciences and Social Sciences* 56 (2001): S365–S373.

15. C. A. Reyes-Ortiz, H. Ayele, T. Mulligan, D. V. Espino, I. M. Berges, and K. S. Markides, "Higher Church Attendance Predicts Lower Fear of Falling in Older Mexican-Americans," *Aging and Mental Health* 10, no. 1 (2006): 13–18.

16. Murray and Lopez, *The Global Burden of Disease*, cited in *British Medical Journal* (2002).

17. R. G. Cumming, G. Salked, M. Thomas, and G. Szonyi, "Prospective Study of the Impact of Fear of Falling on Activities of Daily Living, SF-36 Scores, and Nursing Home Admission," *Journals of Gerontology, Series A: Biological Sciences and Medical Sciences* 55A (2000): M299–M305.

18. E. L. Idler, "Religious Involvement and the Health of the Elderly: Some Hypotheses and an Initial Test," *Social Forces* 66 (1987): 226–38.

19. E. L.Idler, "Religion, Health, and Nonphysical Senses of Self," *Social Forces*, 74, (1995) 683–704.

20. See the following studies: Y. Leyser, "Stress and Adaptation in Orthodox Jewish Families with a Disabled Child," *American Journal of Orthopsychiatry* 64, no. 3 (1994): 376–85; L. L. Treloar, "Disability, Spiritual Beliefs and the Church: The Experiences of Adults with Disabilities and Family Members," *Journal of Advanced Nursing* 40, no. 5 (2002): 594–603; and M. A. McColl, J. Bickenbach, J. Johnston, et al., "Spiritual Issues Associated with Traumatic-Onset Disability," *Disability & Rehabilitation* 22, no. 12 (2000): 555–64.

21. See the following studies: Z. Simmons, B. A. Bremer, R. A. Robbins, S. M. Walsh, and S. Fischer, "Quality of Life in ALS Depends on Factors Other Than Strength and Physical Function," *Neurology* 55, no. 3 (2000): 388–92; B. Brillhart, "A Study of Spirituality and Life Satisfaction among Persons with Spinal Cord Injury," *Rehabilitation Nursing* 30, no. 1 (2005): 31–34; and D. G. Tate and M. Forchheimer, "Quality of Life, Life Satisfaction, and Spirituality: Comparing Outcomes between Rehabilitation and Cancer Patients," *American Journal of Physical Medicine & Rehabilitation* 81, no. 6 (2002): 400–10.

## Chapter 11: Clinical Applications

1. H. G. Koenig, *Spirituality in Patient Care: Why, How, When, and Why*, 2nd ed. (Philadelphia: Templeton Foundation Press, 2007).

2. See the following studies: O. Oyama and H. G. Koenig, "Religious Beliefs and Practices in Family Medicine," *Archives of Family Medicine* 7 (1998): 431–35; C. D. MacLean, B. Susi, N. Phifer, et al., *Journal of General Internal Medicine* 18 (2003): 38–43; and L. C. Kaldjian, J. F. Jekel, and G. Friedland, End-of-Life Decisions in HIV-Positive Patients: The Role of Spiritual Beliefs," *AIDS* 12, no. 1 (1998): 103–7.

3. G. Fitchett, L. A. Burton, and A. B. Sivan, "The Religious Needs and Resources of Psychiatric Patients," *Journal of Nervous and Mental Disease* 185 (1997): 320–26.

4. On the opportunity of seeing a chaplain, see K. J. Flannelly, K. Galek, and G. F. Handzo, "To What Extent Are the Spiritual Needs of Hospital Patients

Being Met?" *International Journal of Psychiatry in Medicine* 35, no. 3 (2005): 319–23. Regarding the problem of health-care professionals in addressing spiritual needs, see the following studies: J. T. Chibnall and C. A. Brooks, "Religion in the Clinic: The Role of Physician Beliefs," *Southern Medical Journal* 94 (2001): 374–79; F. A. Curlin, M. H. Chin, S. A. Sellergren, C. J. Roach, and J. D. Lantos, "The Association of Physicians' Religious Characteristics with Their Attitudes and Self-Reported Behaviors Regarding Religion and Spirituality in the Clinical Encounter," *Medical Care* 44 (2006): 446–53; and D. E. King and B. J. Wells, "End-of-Life Issues and Spiritual Histories," *Southern Medical Journal* 96 (2003): 391–93.

5. P. A. Clark, M. Drain, and M. P. Malone, "Addressing Patients' Emotional and Spiritual Needs," *Joint Commission Journal on Quality and Safety* 29 (2003): 659–70.

6. H. G. Koenig, "Religious Beliefs and Practices of Hospitalized Medically Ill Older Adults," *International Journal of Geriatric Psychiatry* 13 (1998): 213–24.

7. Concerning patients with lung cancer, see G. A. Silvestri, S. Knittig, J. S. Zoller, et al., "Importance of Faith on Medical Decisions Regarding Cancer Care," *Journal of Clinical Oncology* 21 (2003): 1379–82. Concerning patients with lung disease, see J. Ehman, B. Ott, T. Short, R. Ciampa, and J. Hansen-Flaschen, "Do Patients Want Physicians to Inquire about Their Spiritual or Religious Beliefs If They Become Gravely Ill?" *Archives of Internal Medicine* 159 (1999): 1803–6. On end-of-life situations, see B. Lo, D. Ruston, L. Kates, et al., "Discussing Religious and Spiritual Issues at the End of Life: A Practical Guide for Physicians," *Journal of the American Medical Association* 287, no. 6 (2002): 749–54. Finally, regarding patients from various religions, see Koenig, *Spirituality in Patient Care: Why, How, When, and Why*, 2nd ed., chap. 13.

8. Concerning Christian Scientists, see R. Swan, "Faith Healing, Christian Science, and the Medical Care of Children," *New England Journal of Medicine* 302 (1983): 1639–41. Concerning fundamentalist Christians, see D. Biebel and H. G. Koenig, *New Light on Depression: Help and Hope for the Depressed and Those Who Love Them* (New York: Zondervan/HarperCollins, 2004).

9. Joint Commission for the Accreditation of Hospital Organizations. See http://www.jointcommission.org/AccreditationPrograms/Hospitals/Standards/FAQs/Provision+of+Care/Assessment/Spiritual_Assessment.htm (last revised January 1, 2004; last accessed December 28, 2007).

10. Adapted from H. G. Koenig, "An 83-Year-Old Woman with Chronic Illness and Strong Religious Beliefs, *Journal of the American Medical Association* 288, no. 4 (2002): 487–93; and first presented in Koenig, *Spirituality in Patient Care: Why, How, When, and Why*, 2nd ed.

11. J. L. Kristeller, M. Rhodes, L. D. Cripe, and V. Sheets, "Oncologist Assisted Spiritual Intervention Study (OASIS): Patient Acceptability and Initial Evidence of Effects," *International Journal of Psychiatry in Medicine* 35 (2005): 329–47.

12. Ibid., 333.

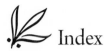 Index

Afghanistan war, 31
African Americans
    alcohol use and, 61
    diabetes and, 122, 124
    disability and, 150
    drug use and, 61–62
    hypertension and, 43, 98, 100–101,
        104–5, 107
    life satisfaction and, 57, 79–80
    religion and, 130, 137, 139, 185
afterlife, 11, 77, 101–2
aging, 5, 29–31, 120, 140
*Aging and God: Spiritual Paths to Mental
    Health* (Koenig), 188
Agrawal, M., 116
Ai, A. L., 118
Akerlof, George, 31
alcohol use, 47–49, 58–61
Alexander, C. N., 142
Al-Kandari, Y. Y., 102
altruism, 9, 49–52, 57, 65–67, 76
Alzheimer's disease, 6, 30, 44, 120–21
*American Journal of Geriatric Psychiatry,*
    179
*American Journal of Psychiatry,* 177
*American Journal of Public Health,* 137
Angell, Marcia, 5
anxiety
    behavioral factors and, 49–50
    religion and, 76–78
Association of Professional Chaplains,
    163
astrology, 12, 17
attitudes, of physicians, 25–27
autoimmune disorders, 82
autonomic nervous system, 38, 46
autonomic rhythms, 6

Balboni, T. A., 24, 185
Basil of Caesarea, Saint, 33
behavioral factors. *See also* coping
    behavior
    anxiety and, 49–50
    depression and, 49
    health and, 48–52, 113–28
    immune system and, 48–49
    mental health and, 50–52
    religion and, 6, 57–65
    spirituality and, 13
beliefs, 19, 57, 116–17, 170. *See also* religion
Benjamins, M. R., 150
Berman, E., 79
Bernanke, Ben, 31
Bernardi, L., 107
*Better Homes and Gardens,* 52
Bible, 55, 72, 98, 111, 142
bipolar disorder, 43
birth rates, 28, 30
Blazer, D. G., 175
*Blind Faith: The Unholy Alliance of
    Religion and Medicine* (Sloan, R.), 190
blood pressure
    confounding variables and, 119
    coping behavior and, 100–101
    mind-body connection and, 37, 42–43
    psychological factors and, 96–97
    religion and, 97–108
    Transcendental Meditation (TM) and,
        104, 107
    well-being and, 100, 124
Blumenthal, J. A., 41
Boehnlein, J. K., 189
*The Boy in the Plastic Bubble,* 82
Braam, A. W., 178
brain activity, 51

Brown, K. W., 44
Brown, S. L., 50
Brummet, B. H., 47
Buchanan, James M., 31
Buddhism, 16
Burns, Scott, 30–32
Bush, George W., 32
Butts, C. O., III, 60
bypass surgery, 41, 45, 117

CAD. *See* coronary artery disease
cancer
 confounding variables and, 126–28
 coping behavior and, 56, 124, 129
 depression and, 72
 endocrine system and, 39
 marital status and, 48
 metastatic, 6, 82
 mind-body connection and, 44–45
 non-Hodgkin's lymphoma, 40
 patients, 24
 religion and, 77–78, 124–27
cardiac surgery, 6, 117–19
cardiovascular system
 clinical trials and, 104–8
 epidemiological studies and, 97–102
 experimental studies and, 103–4
 health behaviors and, 108–11
 marital status and, 100
 mind-body connection and, 47–48
 psychological factors and, 38
 religion and, 96–112
caregivers, 41, 44, 72, 80
Carlson, L. E., 91
CASA. *See* National Center on
 Addiction and Substance Abuse
Castillo-Richmond, A., 107
catecholamine, 39
Catholic Ascension Health Care, 35
cellular immunity, 85–92
Center for Medicare and Medicaid
 Services, 29
chaplains, 25, 60, 157, 163–64
charitable giving, 51, 66, 91
Chi, D. S., 91
clinical applications, 19, 23–25, 156–71,
 194
clinical trials, 104–8, 116–17, 132
cognitive function
 dementia and, 120–22
 depression and, 69
 disability and, 149

mind-body connection and, 40, 47
coherence, sense of, 39
Colantonio, A., 119
*A Coming Generational Storm* (Kotlikoff
 and Burns), 30–32
Comstock, G. W., 179
confounding variables
 blood pressure and, 119
 cancer and, 126–28
 depression and, 73
 explanatory variables v., 130–33
 immune system and, 86
 longevity and, 136, 142–43
 mortality and, 134, 137–40, 149–50
congestive heart failure, 42, 71
Contrada, R. J., 118, 144
coping behavior
 blood pressure and, 100–101
 cancer and, 56, 124, 129
 coronary artery disease (CAD) and,
  116–19
 endocrine system and, 92
 heart disease and, 113, 144
 immune system and, 86, 87, 90, 91
 mental health and, 70, 72, 77, 78, 80, 81
 perceptions of health and, 153
 prayer and, 55–56
 religious coping, 12, 54–56, 148, 156,
  164, 170, 172
 stress and, 166–67
 young persons and, 154–55
coronary artery disease (CAD), 6,
 41–42, 48, 113–19
cortisol, 39, 46–47, 49, 52, 92–95
cosmic consciousness, 13
costs, of health-care, 5, 28–32
crime, 59–60
crisis, in health-care, 4, 21–22, 29, 33–35
cross-sectional studies, 76–77, 79, 81
CSI-MEMO, 161, 166
Curlin, F. A., 26–27
Cutler, S. J., 56
cytotoxic cells, 38, 83, 86, 88–89

*Dallas Morning News,* 30
Davidson, K., 43
Davidson, R. J., 84
Dawal, A. K., 116
debate, on health and religion, 9–20
Dedert, E. A., 93
deficit spending, 31–32
delinquency, 59–60

dementia, 40, 120–22
demographic changes, 28–30
Denton, Melinda, 10
depression
  behavioral factors and, 49
  cancer and, 72
  cognitive function and, 69
  confounding variables and, 73
  disability and, 45, 70–71, 147
  mind-body connection and, 38,
    40–42, 44–45
  mortality and, 69
  religion and, 68–73, 81
  stress and, 71–72
diabetes
  marital status and, 122
  mind-body connection and, 40, 47
  religion and, 100, 115, 122–24
  well-being and, 122–23
diet, 6, 108–10
disability
  African Americans and, 150
  cognitive function and, 149
  depression and, 45, 70–71, 147
  elderly and, 149–52
  marital status and, 149, 151
  physical, 146–55
divorce, 62–63, 67
drug use
  African Americans and, 61–62
  mind-body connection and, 48
  religion and, 58–59, 61–62

education, medical, 24
elderly persons, disability and, 149–52
endocrine system
  cancer and, 39
  coping behavior, 92
  psychological factors and, 39
  psychosocial factors and, 49,
    51–52
  religion and, 82, 92–95
  social factors and, 46–47
  well-being and, 90
epidemiological studies, 97–102
Epstein-Barr virus, 39
ethics, 58–59, 169
exercise, 6, 110–11
existential concerns, 18
Existential Well-Being Scale, 123
experimental studies, 103–4
explanatory variables, 130–33

FACIT-sp. See Functional Assessment
    of Chronic Illness Therapy Spiritual
    Well-Being Scale
faith. See religion
Faith and Mental Health (Koenig), 189
faith communities, 33–36, 62, 154, 159–
    60, 165–66
The Faith Factor (Matthews), 189
family, 13, 58
fear of falling, 152
Fenix, J. B., 72
Ferraro, K. F., 151
fight-or-flight response, 96
fMRI. See functional magnetic
    resonance imaging
Fontana, A., 178
Forman, T. A., 59
Freedman, M., 121
Friedlander, Y., 109, 114
Functional Assessment of Chronic
    Illness Therapy Spiritual Well-Being
    Scale (FACIT-sp), 79, 90
functional magnetic resonance imaging
    (fMRI), 51

Gencoz, T., 62
George, L. K., 187
The Gerontologist, 176
Gillum, R. F., 101
God, Faith and Health (Levin), 189
Goldbourt, U., 114, 180
Gopinath, N., 115
Greening, L., 75
growth hormone, 92–95
Gupta, R., 115

Hall, D. E., 136
Hamilton Depression Rating Scale, 90
Handbook of Religion and Health
    (Koenig), 54, 59, 113, 189
Handbook of Religion and Mental Health
    (Koenig), 189
Harinath, K., 106
Harner, S. D., 84
Harris, Mrs.
  immune system and, 82
  longevity and, 129
  mental health and, 68
  religion and, 3–4, 7, 54, 156–57
Heal Thyself: Spirituality, Medicine
    and the Distortion of Christianity
    (Shuman), 190

*The Healing Connection* (Koenig), 193
*The Healing Power of Faith* (Koenig), 189
health. *See also* mental health
  behavioral factors and, 48–52, 113–28
  longevity and, 28
  marital status and, 45, 47
  ministries, 33–35
  perceptions of, 153–54
  psychological factors and, 38–45
  psychosocial factors and, 48–52
  public, 6, 28
  religion and, 4–5, 9–12, 23–24, 54–67
  social factors and, 45–48
  spirituality and, 4–5, 9–10, 12–13
Health Care Congress, 28
health-care
  costs of, 5, 28–32
  crisis, 4, 21–22, 29, 33–35
  partnerships, 33–36
  policy, 23–24
  spirituality and, 23–25, 172–73
heart disease, 113, 144
Helm, H. M., 181
Hemingway, H., 47
hepatitis B, 38
Hill, A. B., 132
Hill, Peter C., 14
Hill, R. D., 121
Hill, T. D., 182
Hinderliter, A. L., 100
Hispanics, 61
HIV/AIDS
  immune system and, 6, 82, 85
  mind-body connection and, 40
  religion and, 64, 80, 86–87, 93, 95
Hoge Intrinsic Religiosity Scale, 71–72
Holman, C. D., 135
Holtz-Eakin, Douglas, 28
hope, mental health and, 74, 78–81
hostility, 38, 40–43, 48, 91, 94–95
Hufford, David J., 15–16
humanism, 9–10, 13, 17, 20
Hummer, R. A., 127, 139, 182
humoral immunity, 83–85
Hunler, O. S., 62
Hunter, K. I., 50
hypertension
  African Americans and, 43, 98,
    100–101, 104–5, 107
  mind-body connection and, 41,
    42–43
hypothalamic-pituitary-adrenal axis, 38

Idler, E. L., 149, 153, 181
IL-6. *See* interleukin 6
immune system
  behavioral factors and, 48–49
  cellular immunity and, 85–92
  confounding variables and, 86
  coping behavior and, 86, 87, 90, 91
  HIV/AIDS and, 6, 82, 85
  humoral immunity and, 83–85
  infection and, 43–44
  psychological factors and, 38–40
  psychosocial factors and, 39
  religion and, 82–92
  social factors and, 46
  Transcendental Meditation (TM)
    and, 95
Independent Sector, 66
infection, 43–44
Ingram, D. D., 101
interleukin 6 (IL-6), 38, 39–40, 89–90
*International Journal of Psychiatry in
  Medicine,* 180–81, 186
Internet resources, 191–92
Iraq war, 31, 154
Ironson, Gail, 80, 87, 95, 183
Ironson-Woods Spirituality/
  Religiousness Index, 93
*Is Religion Good For Your Health?*
  (Koenig), 188

Jacobson, C. M., 90
JCAHO. *See* Joint Commission for
  the Accreditation of Hospital
  Organizations
Jiang, W., 42
John of the Cross, Saint, 16–17
Johnson, B. R., 59
Joint Commission for the Accreditation
  of Hospital Organizations
  (JCAHO), 159, 162
Jolliffe, J. A., 134
*Journal of Geriatric Psychiatry,* 186
*Journal of Nervous and Mental Disease,*
  179
Journal of the American Medical
  Association, 187

Kabat-Zinn, Jon, 91
Kamei, T., 88
Kark, J. D., 181
Kasl, S. V., 120
Kaufman, Y., 121

Kelley-Moore, J. A., 151
Kennedy, G. J., 177
Kesselring, A., 56
Kim, K. H., 110
Kimura, H., 88
King, D. E., 123
Koenig, Harold G.
  *Aging and God: Spiritual Paths to Mental Health,* 188
  *American Journal of Geriatric Psychiatry,* 179
  *American Journal of Psychiatry,* 177, 178
  *Faith and Mental Health,* 190
  *The Gerontologist,* 176
  *Handbook of Religion and Health,* 54, 59, 113, 189
  *Handbook of Religion and Mental Health,* 189
  *The Healing Connection,* 193
  *The Healing Power of Faith,* 189
  *International Journal of Psychiatry in Medicine,* 181–82, 186
  *Is Religion Good For Your Health?,* 188
  *Journal of Geriatric Psychiatry,* 186
  *Journal of Nervous and Mental Disease,* 179
  *Journal of the American Medical Association,* 187
  *The Link Between Religion and Health,* 190
  *Religion, Health and Aging,* 188
  *Southern Medical Journal,* 182, 187
  *Spirituality in Patient Care,* 156, 191, 193
Kogan, S. M., 61
kosher diet, 109
Kotlikoff, Laurence J., 30–32
Krause, N., 78–79, 101
Kristeller, J. L., 167, 184
Krupski, T. L., 79
Kune, G. A., 126

Larson, D. B., 185
Lee, M. S., 94
Levin, J. S., 177, 186, 188, 189
Lewis, S. C., 43
life satisfaction
  African Americans and, 57, 79–80
  mental health and, 78–79
  mind-body connection and, 50
  religion and, 125, 148
Linden, W., 135

*The Link Between Religion and Health* (Koenig), 190
Linn, M. W., 50
Lipitor, 134, 136
longevity
  confounding variables and, 136, 142–43
  health and, 28
  marital status and, 140
  prayer and, 142–44
  religion and, 6, 9, 129–45
  stroke and, 140
  Transcendental Meditation (TM) and, 142
Loyola, Ignatius, 16
Lutgendorf, S. K., 89, 183
Luther, Martin, 16
Lutheran Advocate Health Care, 35
lymphocytic leukemia, 40
lymphoproliferative responses, 39

macrophage activity, 39
marital status
  cancer and, 48
  cardiovascular system and, 100
  diabetes and, 122
  disability and, 149, 151
  divorce and, 62–63, 67
  health and, 45, 47
  longevity and, 140
  religion and, 62
Marmot, M., 47
Masters, K. S., 103, 183
Matthews, D. A., 144, 189
McClain, C. S., 75
McClain-Jacobson, C., 80
McClelland, David C., 83–84
McCullough, Michael E., 133, 134, 135, 186
McEwen, Bruce, 38
meaning, search for, 13, 18, 74–75, 147
Medicaid, 28, 29
medical education, 24
Medicare, 28, 29, 31–33, 34
medicine, in 21st century, 21–36
meditation, 11. *See also* Transcendental Meditation
Melamed, S., 40
meningococcal bacterium, 38
mental health
  behavioral factors and, 50–52
  coping behavior and, 70, 72, 77, 78, 80, 81
  hope and, 74, 78–81

life satisfaction and, 78–79
religion and, 55–56, 68–81
spirituality and, 14, 18, 19–20, 22
metabolic system, 38
metastatic cancer, 6, 82
methodology, 20, 22–23, 137
Miller, William R., 22
mind-body connection
blood pressure and, 37, 42–43
cancer and, 44–45
cardiovascular system and, 47–48
cognitive function and, 40, 47
depression and, 38, 40–42, 44–45
diabetes and, 40, 47
drug use and, 48
HIV/AIDS and, 40
hypertension and, 41, 42–43
life satisfaction and, 50
mortality and, 50–51
stress and, 37–49
stroke and, 41, 43
mindfulness, 84–85, 91–92, 95, 142
Ming, E. E., 42–43
ministries, for health, 33–35
Moberg, D. O., 174
mobility, 110, 123, 130, 137–38
Moll, J., 51
mononucleosis, 39
Montambo, L., 116
morality, 11, 17
morbidity, 41–42, 47–48, 111
mortality
confounding variables and, 134, 137–40, 149–50
depression and, 69
mind-body connection and, 50–51
religion and, 141, 144–45
Mueller, P. S., 187
Mullins, L. C., 62–63
musculoskeletal pain, 55
myocardial infarction, 41, 113–17, 135
myocardial ischemia, 42, 115–17

National Center on Addiction and Substance Abuse (CASA), 60
National Institutes of Health (NIH), 22–23
National Institutes of Mental Health, 70
Native Americans, 61
natural killer cells (NK), 38–39, 48–49, 83, 88–89

networks, social, 45–46, 48, 66, 86–87, 140
Neumann, J. K., 91
neurological function, 40, 47, 70
New England Journal of Medicine, 5, 38
Newlin, K., 122, 124
NIH. See National Institutes of Health
nirvana, 11, 16
Nishino Breathing Method, 88
NK cells. See natural killer cells
non-Hodgkin's lymphoma, 40
norepinephrine, 39
nursing homes, 29–30, 69, 152, 159, 166

OASIS, 168, 184–85
Oman, D., 50, 125
orthodoxy, 12, 75, 109, 114–15
Oxman, T. E., 117, 180

Palouzian and Ellison's Spiritual Well-Being Scale, 122, 124
Pargament, Ken I., 14, 181, 188
Park, N. S., 150
partnerships, health care and, 33–36
Paul-Labrador, M., 106
peace, inner, 13–14, 17
perceptions, of health, 153–54
Perk, G., 108
Peteet, J., 191
physical disability, 146–55
physicians
attitudes of, 25–27
prayer and, 27, 164–65, 169
pneumococcal bacterium, 38
policy, for health care, 23–24
political forces, 32–33
positive psychology, 10, 14, 18, 22
Powell, L. H., 187
Pratt, L. A., 41
prayer
coping behavior and, 55–56
longevity and, 142–44
physicians and, 27, 164–65, 169
Progressive Muscle Relaxation, 104–6
Propst, L. R., 176
prosocial activities, 65–67, 76
Psychiatry and Religion: The Convergence of Mind and Spirit (Boehnlein), 189
psychological factors
blood pressure and, 96–97
cardiovascular system and, 38
endocrine system and, 39

health and, 38–45
immune system and, 38–40
religion and, 53
*The Psychology of Religion and Coping*
(Pargament), 188
psychology, positive. *See* positive
psychology
psychoneuroimmunology, 5, 38, 190
psychosocial factors
endocrine system and, 49, 51–52
health and, 48–52
immune system and, 39
stress and, 82–83
psychosomatic medicine, 5
public health, 6, 28
purpose, 13–14, 18, 74

Qigong, 88, 94
quality of life, 9, 24–25

Raikkonen, K., 40
Rammohan, A., 56
reincarnation, 16
religion
African Americans and, 130, 137, 139,
185
alcohol use and, 47–49, 58–61
anxiety and, 76–78
behavioral factors and, 6, 57–65
blood pressure and, 97–108
cancer and, 77–78, 124–27
cardiovascular system and, 96–112
crime/delinquency and, 59–60
depression and, 68–73, 81
diabetes and, 100, 115, 122–24
divorce and, 62–63, 67
drug use and, 58–59, 61–62
endocrine system and, 82, 92–95
health and, 4–5, 9–12, 23–24, 54–67
HIV/AIDS and, 64, 80, 86–87, 93, 95
immune system and, 82–92
life satisfaction and, 125, 148
longevity and, 6, 9, 129–45
marital status and, 62
mental health and, 55–56, 68–81
mortality and, 141, 144–45
as prosocial agent, 65–67, 76
psychological factors and, 53
sexual promiscuity and, 63–64
spirituality and, 14–20
stress, 67, 113–28, 166–67
stroke and, 119–20

suicide and, 68–69, 74–76
venereal disease and, 64–65
well-being and, 78–79
*Religion and Psychiatric Disorders for
DSM-V* (Peteet), 191
*Religion and the Clinical Practice of
Psychology* (Shafranske), 188
*Religion, Health and Aging* (Koenig), 188
*Religion in Aging and Health* (Levin), 188
religiosity, 11, 12
religious coping. *See* coping behavior
Religious Orientation Scale, 103
Religious Well-Being Scale, 123
research, rigorous requirements of,
18–20
Rew, L., 186
Reyes-Ortiz, C. A., 152
rheumatoid arthritis, 91
Ringdal, G., 125
risk-taking, 59, 64–65, 127
Rosal, M. C., 46

sacred, search for, 11, 14–15, 17
Salsman, J. M., 78
Samuelson, Paul A., 31
Sanua, V. D., 184
Sapolsky, R. M., 47
Saroglou, 66
SCHIP, 29
schizophrenia, 56, 81
Schneider, Ed, 29
Schwartz, C., 50, 66
*Science*, 29
Scott, J., 77
sexual promiscuity, 63–64
sexually transmitted diseases, 64–65
Shafranske, E. P., 188
Shuman, J. J., 190
Silvestri, G. A., 184
Sloan, J. S., 186
Sloan, R. P., 190
Smith, Christian, 10
Smith, G. D., 134
Smith, T. B., 70–71
smoking, 3, 6, 47–49, 111–12
Sobal, J., 110
social factors
endocrine system and, 46–47
health and, 45–48
immune system and, 46
networks, 45–46, 48, 66, 86–87, 140
Social Security, 31–33

somatization, 50
*Southern Medical Journal,* 182, 187
spiritual history, 160–64, 166–69
spiritual needs, 18, 23–26, 156–60, 172–73
Spiritual Well-Being Scale, 122–23
spirituality
  behavioral factors and, 13
  health and, 4–5, 9–10, 12–13
  health care and, 23–25, 172–73
  mental health and, 14, 18, 19–20, 22
  religion and, 14–20
*Spirituality in Patient Care* (Koenig), 156,
  191, 193
Stefano, G. B., 52
Steffen, P. R., 100, 183
Steinman, K. J., 61
stem-cell research, 28–29
Stoppelbein, L., 75
Strawbridge, W. J., 110, 137, 139, 181
stress
  coping behavior and, 166–67
  depression and, 71–72
  mind-body connection and, 37–49
  psychosocial factors and, 82–83
  religion and, 67, 113–28, 166–67
Stress Education Control, 105–6
stroke
  longevity and, 140
  mind-body connection and, 41, 43
  religion and, 119–20
  Transcendental Meditation (TM) and,
  107, 112
suicide, 68–69, 74–76
Sullivan, M. D., 42
supernatural, 12, 15, 17, 20, 37
support
  emotional, 50, 159
  social, 5, 13–14, 18, 23–24, 34–35, 45–48,
    51, 53, 56–57, 67, 78, 87, 93–94, 100–
    101, 122, 127, 131–33, 141, 148, 170
  spiritual, 19, 24–25, 27, 55, 56, 75, 158
  systems, 166
Sussman, S., 61
syphilis, 64

Tartaro, J., 94, 103
tautology, 18
Teresa, Mother, 84
Teresa of Avila, Saint, 16

terrorist attacks, 54–55
theology, 7
*Time,* 98–99
TM. *See* Transcendental Meditation
transcendence, 13, 15–16, 17
Transcendental Meditation (TM)
  blood pressure and, 104, 107
  CAD and, 116
  cortisol and, 92
  immune system and, 95
  longevity and, 142
  stroke and, 107, 112
Travolta, John, 82
Tully, J., 184
tumor necrosis factor, 39
Type A personality, 41

United Nations, 30

vaccinations, 38, 44
values, 13, 18
Van Gelder, B. M., 47
Van Ness, P. H., 120
Van Olphen, J., 122
Van Tubergen, F., 74
Vaupel, James W., 129
venereal disease, 64–65
volunteering, 50–51, 65–67

*Wall Street Journal,* 28
Wallace, J. M., 59
well-being
  blood pressure and, 100, 124
  diabetes and, 122–23
  endocrine system and, 90
  religion and, 78–79
White, H. R., 61
Wilson, R. S., 40
Wink, P., 77
Woods, T. E., 86
workshops, 194

Yeager, D. M., 90, 94, 102, 121, 142
Yelsma, P., 116

Zamarra, J. W., 116
Zhang, J., 40
Zimmerman, M. A., 61